*H*ow to Stay Out of The Doctor's Office

An Encyclopedia For Alternative Healing

*H*ow to Stay Out of The Doctor's Office

An Encyclopedia For Alternative Healing

"HOW TO STAY OUT OF THE DOCTOR'S OFFICE is a comprehensive guide to a new method of improving health through nutrition and supplements. I recommend it highly."

- Miriam Ershkowitz, Ph.D., Professor of Public Health Management, Public Health Consultant

Dr. Edward M. Wagner
with
Sylvia Goldfarb

Instant Improvement, Inc.

How to Stay Out of the Doctor's Office
An Encyclopedia for Alternative Healing
Dr. Edward M. Wagner with Sylvia Goldfarb
Copyright © 1992 by Edward M.Wagner

Published by Instant Improvement, Inc., 210 East 86th Street, New York, New York 10028.

Printed in the United States of America

Second Printing 1993

Library of Congress Cataloging-in-Publication Data

Wagner, Edward M.
    How to stay out of the doctor's office : an encyclopedia for alternative healing / Edward M. Wagner with Sylvia Goldfarb.
      p. cm.
    ISBN 0-941683-18-4
    1. Alternative medicine--Encyclopedias. 2. Diet therapy--Encyclopedias. 3. Dietary supplements--Encyclopedias.
I. Goldfarb, Sylvia. II. Title.
R733.W3 1992
615.5'03--dc20   92-32307

Important

You will find Dr. Wagner's advice extremely valuable in following your personal physician's recommendations. The information provided is for your better health. However, any decision you make involving the treatment of an illness should include your family doctor. Naturally, since individual metabolisms vary, not everyone can experience identical or optimum results. Before beginning any program of exercise, please consult your physician.

Contents

INTRODUCTION

I DIDN'T HAVE LONG TO LIVE IF FAMILY HISTORY IN-
dicated longevity. I was a well-respected architect with a promising future, but having lost both parents and a brother to heart disease,
my prospects for a long life were rather bleak.

I realized that I had to do something drastic to improve my chance
for survival, and since orthodox medicine had not helped my family,
I started to search for a method to increase my opportunity for a long
and healthy life. Due to the nature of my work, I knew there was
more than one way to solve a problem. I applied my architectural
background and scientific way of thinking to learn how the body
functions.

As I began to understand human biochemistry, I became convinced the only way an individual can maintain health is by eliminating all negativity entering the body. This includes drugs, alcohol,
smoking, processed and refined foods and negative thoughts. The
orthodoxy addresses symptoms rather than causes, and eventually
the original symptoms return.

The first thing I learned was that my diet, drinking habits and
attitude were terrible. My usual routine after work was to have a
few drinks and pick up dinner at a fast-food restaurant. I changed
my diet, stopped drinking and experimented with vitamins, minerals, imagery and positive affirmations.

My friends and colleagues noticed such a difference about me
that they started to ask me for advice. After a period of self-study,
I decided to further my education and took formal courses in biochemistry, nutrition, vitamin and mineral therapy, herbal remedies
and iridology (a diagnostic method of interpreting the iris).

I left my job as an architect and did consultations in health food
stores and in Chiropractors' offices. In 1984 I received a Doctor's
Degree in Nutrition from the American Nutritional Medical Association, and I have been advising patients and lecturing full-time
since then. My colleagues are Chiropractors, Doctors of Osteopathy,
Nutritional Medical Doctors, Naturopathic Physicians, Homeopaths
and other nutritionists.

Patients seek my advice after undergoing years of unsuccessful
medical treatment. By the time they reach me, they are convinced

that orthodox medical treatment is not curing their ailments. Many have friends who were helped by alternative modalities that led to natural healing processes.

A large percentage of my practice is devoted to helping people with digestive disturbances and problems with weight control such as a 33-year-old male suffering from constipation, obesity and fatigue, who was referred to me by his mother. After questioning him about whether he suffered from bloating, gas or indigestion following consumption of certain foods, I discovered he could not metabolize carbohydrates and that toxins that should have been eliminated from his body were backing up into his system. I suggested he eliminate all processed foods, processed sugars and refined carbohydrates and gave him a series of nutritional treatments designed to eliminate constipation and activate his normal bowel movements. After six days, his fatigue disappeared and normal bowel movements returned. Toxins were eliminated, he lost weight and now feels mentally and physically better.

People with high blood pressure often have problems with side effects from medication prescribed by their doctors. A 59-year-old male who had been taking diuretics and heart calcium blockers felt lethargic and suffered feelings of spaciness. He was also overweight. I suggested he stop eating all carbohydrates, both refined and complex, and go on a high protein diet, which has a natural diuretic effect. I recommended supplements including Vitamin C, B6 and an herbal combination that would aid his body to rid itself of excess fluids, thereby bringing his blood pressure down. His blood pressure has remained at 128/72.

Cancer patients have exhausted immune systems from the effects of chemotherapy, radiation, surgery and other drugs. Treatments can kill the cancer cells, but if the cells are not expunged from the body, they can cause a poisonous reaction similar to gangrene. This fact is not addressed by orthodox medical practitioners.

A year after undergoing a lumpectomy and chemotherapy for breast cancer, a woman developed cancer in the opposite breast with lymph node involvement. Following radiation therapy, blood tests showed cancer cells were still in her body, proving that chemotherapy was ineffective. She believed that radiation and chemotherapy had not helped the cancer to vanish. She started nutritional therapy and also took five coffee enemas a day. She also took a series of nutritional supplements consisting mainly of pancreatic enzymes, which destroy viruses. Most cancer patients have a depleted supply of this enzyme. In order to further enhance her immune system, specific supplements were given to stimulate her adrenal and thymus glands.

Radiation therapy had caused burns on her breast. These were treated with castor oil packs, and soon disappeared. I taught her how to employ positive imagery, which had a phenomenal effect on eliminating her negative interpretation of life. She is now symptom free and her prognosis is excellent.

After years of clinical practice, I have determined most ailments can be reversed by my methods unless there is severe anatomical damage. Chronic ailments usually do not improve when treated by orthodox allopathic practitioners since symptoms are treated and causes are not addressed.

Medication treats symptoms, disregarding the reason behind them. Medicine works by blocking the effects of the illness, but it does not rebuild diseased tissue. Eventually this blocking system causes side effects on other parts of the body often leading to iatro- genic (doctor induced) illness. For instance, medication for hypertension causes retention of uric acid which can lead to gout. Cholesterol-lowering drugs also stop absorption of the fat-soluble vitamins A, E, D, and K. Medication for ulcers works by slowing or stopping acid production in the stomach, which in turn stops the breakdown of protein type foods by hydrochloric acid. Then the body cannot absorb essential fatty acids from protein, and other digestive disturbances appear, including colitis, irritable bowel syndrome and diverticulitis. Patients are given medication containing ingredients which their bodies are not deficient in, when instead it would be better to give them the nutrients in which they are deficient.

My method is to find the deficiency that allowed the tissue to deteriorate to the point of causing disease. Then tissue is rebuilt by supplying vitamins, minerals, amino acids, essential fatty acids and correct diet. Natural healing is inexpensive, non-toxic, has a high percentage of cure rate and is at any individual's grasp. Alternative modalities can help approximately 75 percent of people who follow the recommended diet and supplements. Actually 90 percent could be helped if they adhered strictly to the recommended regime.

The average person is unaware of this other way to alleviate illness outside of orthodox medical treatment. An individual should have freedom of choice to select conventional or alternative therapy for disease and illness. This book, which encompasses alternative modalities, can allow uninformed patients another choice besides orthodox medicine.

Most other books of this type consist of all sorts of information on only one condition and contain page after page of technical information that most readers just skim through. Here, in one book, is an easy reference of non-toxic methods for a variety of ailments. Chapters are short and information is to the point, with material presented in an uncomplicated fashion describing causes, conventional treatment, problems with conventional treatment and alternative natural modalities. The conditions described in this book are the ones about which I am most often consulted. I chose not to address acute infectious diseases because they can be treated satisfactorily by allopathic medicine since treatment is on a short-term basis.

If orthodox medicine was working, the population would not turn to alternative healing. Most of the grim statistics show orthodox medicine has failed, especially in the war against cancer. But the battle for patients' rights and free selection of medical therapy has just begun.

Medical attention should definitely be sought in all emergencies when danger is imminent, such as accidents, high fever, stroke or heart attack. Because everyone is different, the information in this book is not given as medical advice and should not be used for self diagnosing or self medicating. Rather, it is of a general nature to educate people that there are choices in health care.

When using supplements in therapeutic doses, periodic blood tests should be performed to insure that blood levels are normal. After the condition is gone, check with your nutritionist or holistic physician for maintenance doses.

ACNE

DEFINITION

Acne is an inflammatory disease of the skin, especially the face, arising from obstruction of the sebaceous glands. It occurs most frequently among teenagers following puberty. If severe degrees of acne are not treated, scar tissue can form in the area.

CAUSES

An overproduction of sebum, a fatty secretion produced by small glands under the skin, causes clogging of the pores, often leading to a bacterial infection. This overproduction of sebum is caused by the intake of foods high in saturated fats or sugars which become saturated fats in the blood. A zinc deficiency will cause enlargement of the sebaceous glands.

Allergies to environmental constituents.

Food allergies.

Allergic reactions to cosmetics.

An overabundance of toxins in the system inundates normal channels of excretion, such as the bowels, urinary tract and lungs. These toxins will then be excreted through the skin and combine with surface bacteria, causing infection.

CONVENTIONAL TREATMENT

Antibiotics to reduce inflammation, such as clindamycin, cleocint or others.

Ultraviolet rays.

Dermabrasion for scars.

Drying agents.

Retin A.

Acutane.

PROBLEMS ASSOCIATED WITH CONVENTIONAL TREATMENT

Acne medicine can cause an imbalance of insulin levels, hormone levels, or blood pressure and neurotransmitter levels. Antibiotics also destroy both good and bad bacteria, leading to an imbalance of the intestinal flora. This can cause a proliferation of yeast in the colon and intestines and can lead to a Candida albicans or fungus infection.

Ultraviolet radiation can lead to skin cancer.

Retin A is an analog of Vitamin A. High doses of Vitamin A have deleterious side effects on the liver. Since Retin A has to be used continually, these patients should be checked periodically for liver damage.

Drying agents have to be controlled carefully because the skin needs a certain amount of oil to keep it flexible and prevent premature aging.

ALTERNATIVE NATURAL REMEDIES

Diet Change

Consumption of foods that interfere with the liver's ability to function properly as a detoxifying organ must be eliminated. These include processed sugars, dairy products, saturated fats and all foods causing the individual to have an allergic reaction. In stubborn cases, allergy testing should be done to determine environmental or dietary allergies.

Eliminate alcohol and medicinal and recreational drugs.

Avoid commercial soft drinks containing brominated vegetable oil.

Pollution Avoidance

Stay away from tobacco smoke. If you are a smoker, stop, and remember that secondary smoke is also harmful to your body. Smoking constricts every blood vessel in the body.

Try to avoid working or being in areas where chemicals are prevalent.

Supplements

Beta carotene A (the healthy skin vitamin), 25,000 I.U. four times daily.

This is pro vitamin A, not an oil-based form. It is water soluble which means the body uses what it needs and eliminates the rest. It does not accumulate in the liver to the degree where it can cause liver dysfunction. The side effect it sometimes has is that the skin, especially on the hands and feet, can take on an orange tint. If this should occur, cut down the amount and within two weeks the skin color will return to normal. Zinc picolinate, 50 mg. two times a day. Zinc helps Vitamin A to be processed through the liver and helps stimulate antibodies to ward off the infectious bacteria on the skin.

Vitamin C (ester C), 1000 mg. four times daily. Ester C is less acidic, more absorbable, more effective and stays in the system longer.

Herbs

Horsetail—tones the skin.

Red clover combination—a blood purifier and cleanser. It also helps the liver remove toxins from the body.

Jojoba.

Dandelion root—a liver cleanser.

Silymarin (milk thistle) aids in the regeneration of liver cells needed to detoxify poisons. It also protects liver cells from further damage.

Amino Acids

L-Cysteine, 500 mg. twice daily on empty stomach, acts as an antioxidant for the skin. Use three times as much Vitamin C (3000mg.) as L-Cysteine to prevent formation of kidney stones.

Local Therapy

Keep the skin clean. Wash with Dr. Bonners soap, available in health food stores, or use a similar product.

Benzoyl peroxide, 5 percent gel, applied to your face at night after washing with non-medicated soap, increases blood flow to your face.

Apply aloe vera gel three times a day. Store it in the refrigerator.

To eliminate acne scarring, apply Vitamin E oil twice daily. Results should be apparent in three months.

To relieve inflammation, rub the inside of a banana peel over the affected areas.

AGING

DEFINITION

A degenerative process of the breakdown of cellular matter. The chronological breakdown is ongoing until death.

CAUSES

The speed at which aging occurs is determined by the induction of toxins into the body. These toxins, derived from chemicals and other adverse matter cause the deterioration of the biochemistry of cellular structure. Substances within the cell derived from basic vitamins, minerals and amino acids are depleted.

In the process of providing energy in the body, a by-product is formed. This by-product, known as free radical production, is what causes the breakdown of cellular matter. Free radicals are composed of extra electrons, which are lost and trying to find a new home. They alight onto other molecules, causing an imbalance of their electrons. This slowly destroys and imbalances the molecular production of energy in that cell.

This process can be slowed or reversed by altering the chemical imbalance. Then new energies are metabolized, causing fresh growth of tissue, bone and other structural forms.

CONVENTIONAL TREATMENT

At this time orthodox medical treatment has nothing to reverse aging.

Cosmetic surgery can temporarily change the outward appearance of a person.

PROBLEMS ASSOCIATED WITH CONVENTIONAL TREATMENT

Any type of surgical procedure carries a certain amount of risk and leaves some residual scar tissue, which is a storage deposit of toxins in the body, specifically bacteria and viruses that tend to accumulate in dead tissue.

ALTERNATIVE NATURAL REMEDIES

Stress Reduction

Stress affects glands and organs to the point of disproportionate production of hormones. When hormones are out of balance, tissues become vulnerable to disease. These natural chemicals strengthen tissues, collagen and protein, and enable your body to rebound from time-caused damages. Stress can change the production of these chemicals that are especially necessary to fend off the never-ending attack of gravity.

Exercise

Exercise is needed for the continued circulation of blood and lymphatic fluid.

Massage

Considered by many to be a luxury, massage has the therapeutic effect of stimulating the lymphatic system, the body's cleansing program.

Diet

Maintain normal weight by properly balancing fats, proteins and carbohydrates. Recommended proportions are: 5 percent fats, 10 percent proteins and 85 percent complex carbohydrates.

Try to eat as much raw food as possible, such as fruit, uncooked vegetables, nuts, seeds and sprouts. The reason is that enzymes are needed to digest food. About half the enzymes are in the food and half in the stomach lining. When food enters the stomach, as part of the digestive process, its enzymes break the food down. This is the beginning of the metabolism of nutrients needed by the body.

Heat used in cooking destroys the living enzymes in the food. Then the stomach is forced to overproduce digestive enzymes from its lining. This overproduction eventually causes a depletion of other enzymes, particularly pancreatic enzymes needed for the destruction of pathogens.

Elimination

Due to the huge amount of toxins in the environment, it is vital to keep all bodily functions working to avoid backup of waste matter. Adequate fluid intake and an abundance of raw foods will insure proper elimination of urine and feces.

Perspiration is one of the best modalities to rid the body of excess toxins. It can be increased by exercising and/or using a steam room or sauna.

Supplements

Antioxident types of vitamins, minerals and amino acids are needed because oxygen used up by metabolism causes the overproduction of free radicals.

Vitamin A, 25,000 I.U. (Beta carotene).

B Complex, 50 mg. twice daily.

Vitamin C, 500 mg. four times daily.

Vitamin E, 400 I.U.

Zinc picolinate, 30 mg.

Selenium, 200 mg.

Glutathione, 300 mg. between meals.

Bee pollen, as directed on label.

Ginseng, as directed on label.

Progestade (for females only) is natural progesterone and a combination of DHEA, an anti-aging natural hormone that the body produces and that can be found in health food stores. Natural progesterone can also be found as an extract of wild Mexican Yam, available in health food stores as an herb. Take as directed on label.

Relaxation

The overexertion of a person's limitations causes tissue breakdown to occur at a faster rate. In addition to getting enough sleep, time should be allotted for a rest period during the day in the form of a nap, meditation or yoga.

AIDS

DEFINITION

AIDS stands for Aquired Immuno Deficiency Syndrome, a condition whereby the immune system cells have been infected with the human immunodeficiency virus. The body can no longer fight off illnesses caused by a virus, bacteria, fungus or other pathogens because the compromised immune system is unable to defend it.

CAUSES

A compromised immune system is caused by a lifestyle deleterious to the well-being and health of the host. In these cases the metabolic system has been abused to such a degree that the virus has no trouble infiltrating the immune system cells. These are antibodies and immunoglobulins such as T-cells, Killer cells, suppressor cells, lymphocytes and phagocytes. The weakness of the immune system is further debilitated by poor diet, lack of exercise, chemicals in food, water and air. In addition, emotional states are generally depressed, especially if homosexual tendencies are present. Our society regards homosexuals as outcasts, an attitude which causes them to be depressed and lowers the immune system. Intravenous drug users and practitioners of unsafe sexual methods are also at risk.

CONVENTIONAL TREATMENT

AZT and DDI

PROBLEMS ASSOCIATED WITH CONVENTIONAL TREATMENT

In the process of attacking the disease, AZT and DDI also destroy bone marrow, which is the center for red blood cell production. Most participants in this therapy get devastating blood problems such as anemia, high or low platelet count and high or low hemoglobin.

Since the immune system is already compromised, other diseases may occur such as pneumocystic pneumonia, Kaposi's Sarcoma and Candida albicans (yeast infections). AZT and DDI depress the immune system (which all drugs do) leaving the host wide open for these diseases to take hold in the body.

ALTERNATIVE NATURAL REMEDIES

Build up and stimulate the immune system to the point of defeating and expelling the virus from the body. This is done by:

Lifestyle Changes

A more positive outlook, controlling emotions and reducing stress.

More Positive Outlook

The patient should accept the fact that he or she has the disease and not deny it. They should state over and over through affirmations that they are not dying from the disease but living with it and are well and not sick. No one has the right to give a human being a death notice. The mind can help a person get better if that person really wants to be cured. There are no incurable diseases, only incurable people.

Controlling Emotions

Learn to say no to things you do not want to do. Have complete control and discipline over your body and mind. Learn that stress is nothing more than the outside world commanding you. When you are in charge of your life and love yourself, everyone will love you too, and you will be content. This will stimulate your immune system.

Reducing Stress

Set limits for yourself and don't go past them. You don't have to conquer the world. No one ever has, and no one ever will. Stress is nothing more than being in a situation you can't handle because you were unable to judge the future. Take care of today, and then work on tomorrow. By then you will know who you are dealing with. Build up your self-esteem by sticking up for your God-given rights, and you will learn to love yourself. Those who love themselves don't care what the world thinks. Their stress levels drop to zero.

Dietary Changes

Eliminate junk food, processed food, sugar and high fat foods.

Eat the following foods:

Organically grown fruits, green vegetables, potatoes, carrots, beets, yams, beans, brown rice, corn and whole grain bread and pasta.

High protein type foods—sea fish (not shellfish), range grown turkey and organic eggs, soft boiled or poached only since high heat destroys the lecithin which protects you from the cholesterol. Lower cooking temperatures also protect the egg against overoxidation, the cause of undue rancidity in the fat.

Plain yogurt, raw certified goat's milk, nuts and seeds.

Shitake and Reishi mushrooms stimulate the immune system and raise the T-cell count.

Adequate Exercise

At least 15 minutes a day of an enjoyable type of aerobic exercise and a half hour walk. If possible try to work out on a mini trampoline, which activates the lymph system and cleanses the system of toxins.

Pollution Avoidance

Avoid industrial chemical pollution, smog, gas emissions on the street and interior pollution such as formaldehyde in rugs and new furniture. Aluminum is toxic and is found in antacids, some medications, pots and pans, tap water, baking soda, aluminum wrap and processed foods. Chlorine in tap water turns to chloroform, a carcinogen, when heated to high temperatures, especially when taking hot baths or showers.

Gas fumes in the house are toxic. They can come from a gas stove that is not properly exhausted. Fumes can seep into the house if an automobile is driven into a garage and the door closed immediately (outgassing).

Supplements

Megadoses of Vitamin C—50,000 to 100,000 mg. a day by intravenous drip for two weeks, followed by a maintenance dose of 5000 mg. a day orally. This should be given until diarrhea occurs, then cut back by 10 percent until it stops.

Vitamin A, fish liver oil and Beta carotene, 50,000 I.U.

Vitamin E, 1200 I.U.

Zinc, 100 mg.

Glutathione, 300 mg.

Cysteine, 1000 mg.

Methionine, 1000 mg.

Acidophilus, 2 billion viable cells each capsule, 5 daily.

Germanium, 500 mg.

Dimethyl glycine, 250 mg.

Garlic, 3000 mg.

Ginseng, 1000 mg.

Egg yolk lecithin, which is similar to AL 721 which the Israeli doctors have used with great success.

These doses are considered megadoses and must be administered by a doctor specializing in nutritional medicine who will consider the degree and length of illness and body weight.

Herbs

Jason Winter's Tea—a cancer fighter.

Echinacea—a natural antibiotic and immune stimulant.

Pau D'Arco—an immune stimulant.

Sun chlorella (blue green algae)—immune stimulant.

Red clover combination—a blood purifier and cleanser.

Silymarin (milk thistle)—regenerates the liver.

Amino Acids

N-Aceytl Cysteine, 600 mg. every other day on empty stomach. The reason for taking this amino acid every other day is that it is a detoxifier for heavy metal poisoning, and an extra day is needed to eliminate the toxins and prevent them from inundating the body.

L-Glutathione, 500 mg. twice daily on empty stomach, stimulates the immune system, eliminates free radicals from the body and slows the oxidation of cellular membranes.

L-Histidine, 500 mg. twice daily on empty stomach, reduces the release of histamine and leukotrines from mast cells which can be inflammatory.

L-Methionine, 500 mg. twice daily on empty stomach, aids in detoxifying environmental pollutants, prevents fat cohesion in the liver and promotes antibody production.

L-Lysine, 500 mg. twice daily on empty stomach, reduces the inflammatory response of antibodies (for autoimmune response).

ALCOHOLISM

DEFINITION

Alcoholism is an addictive condition where an individual has taken up the imbibing of alcoholic substances for the purpose of escaping reality. Alcoholics do not have the wherewithal or knowledge to be able to face reality. The alcohol allows them the luxury of escaping from a past which is tormented, hellish and uncompromising.

CAUSES

Pain

When a mother's and father's demands on the child are opposite to each other and the child chooses a side, he or she pays the price of guilt feelings toward the other parent. These children live in constant pain that they think is normal.

Sugar Imbalance

The energy capacity of the body is basically derived from the conversion of sugar into glucose. Alcohol has the highest sugar content of any food substance. One gram of carbohydrate equals 4 calories. One gram of alcohol equals 7.5 calories. Secondary alcoholics are able to derive sugar from foods such as chocolate, cookies, cake, candy and ice cream.

Some individuals with an abnormally high need for sugar, turn to alcohol, because of its higher caloric content, to replenish their energy capacity. These people are predisposed to craving sugar because of an overproduction of insulin in the pancreas (hyperinsulinism). After metabolizing the glucose in the bloodstream, some insulin is left over. If not utilized, it seeks out carbohydrates which at the moment are not there. This leads to a craving for still more carbohydrates to be broken down by the excess insulin.

If an alcoholic's family lineage is investigated, a parent or grandparent will often be found with a sugar imbalance problem. This may be in the form of diabetes, either juvenile or adult onset, or hypoglycemia.

Social and Psychological

Some people are bored or lonely and frequent bars and consume alcohol to be in the company of others.

CONVENTIONAL TREATMENT

Alcoholics Anonymous.

Drugs such as antabuse.

Counseling.

Clinics.

Behavior Modification.

Anti-depressant medication.

PROBLEMS ASSOCIATED WITH CONVENTIONAL TREATMENT

No conventional treatment deals with the problem of sugar imbalance in the drinker's metabolism. People who attempt to stop drinking and who are not treated for this imbalance can have severe withdrawal symptoms.

Orthodox doctors do not treat through diet or strengthen the immune system. Thus the underlying disease remains dormant, and will erupt and spread throughout the body again.

Alcoholics Anonymous is a wonderful support group, but the refreshments served at the end of the meetings consist of highly sugared donuts and Danish pastries served with coffee, which stimulates the release of glycogen into the bloodstream. This eventually causes blood sugar to drop, leading to an even stronger craving for more alcohol.

ALTERNATIVE NATURAL REMEDIES

Treat the sugar imbalance.

Diet

Eat a high protein, low carbohydrate diet. Protein comes from living creatures such as chicken, turkey, fish, which ounce for ounce, has more protein and less fat than red meat, eggs and dairy products. All carbohydrates eventually convert to glucose, while proteins are metabolized by a different process. By eliminating or lessening carbohydrate intake, insulin production is reduced, thus eliminating the sugar craving. The worst carbohydrates are the simple ones such as candy, cookies, cake, white sugar, sodas, honey, molasses, ice cream and food that has been refined and processed.

Supplements

Alcoholics have a depletion of certain vitamins and enzymes affecting the breakdown of alcohol by the liver. A full dietary regime of vitamins, minerals and amino acids is needed for rebuilding the body after the cessation of drinking. Improperly metabolized sugar causes thickening of blood and displaces oxygen in the blood-stream. This can lead to circulatory problems such as stroke, heart problems, high blood pressure, high cholesterol and atherosclerosis. These supplements help eliminate the craving for alcohol by improving sugar metabolism.

Vitamin B1 (thiamine), 200 mg. twice daily, helps to digest carbohydrates and calm the nervous system.

Chromium picolinate, 200 mcg. three times daily, helps the glucose and insulin to enter the cell by receptor sites which are inactivated in chromium deficient alcoholics.

L-Glutamine, an amino acid, 500 mg. four times daily, between meals helps reduce the craving for alcohol by instilling an amino acid type glucose, which does not need insulin, into the body.

Zinc picolinate, 35 mg. and manganese, 50 mg. twice daily each, are necessary for the chemical breakdown of sugar.

Herbs

Take herbs according to directions on label.

Hops is good for delirium.

Cayenne takes the enlarged blood vessels that appear on the nose, which cause it to have a large reddened appearance, and reduces them.

Valerian, passion flower and skullcap act as sedatives without side effects.

Detoxification

The liver is constantly cleansing the body of all toxins, If it is overburdened with the additional toxins of too much alcohol, it will eventually fail and lead to cirrhosis and untimely death. Therefore, it is extremely important for alcoholics to cleanse the liver.

Chaparral helps remove the residue of alcohol.

Red clover combination is a liver cleanser.

Silymarin (milk thistle) regenerates the cells of the liver.

Uva ursi is a diuretic that helps the kidneys eliminate toxins.

Fiber in the form of psyllium seed husks acts as a bulking agent and helps alleviate constipation.

Fluid intake, at least 8 glasses of liquid daily, preferably in the form of distilled water, keeps the kidneys working which is another way to detoxify the body.

ALLERGY

DEFINITION

An allergy is an inappropriate or harmful immunologic response to a substance which is harmless to most people. The body over-reacts to substances such as foods, drugs, inhalants, pollen, infectious agents or other contaminants. The most common allergies are asthma, hay fever and eczema. Pollen from brightly colored flowers is not as aggravating to allergies as grass, trees or ragweed. Pollen counts are highest on warm sunny days and lowest when it is raining. More pollen is in the air in the morning, and it decreases during the day.

CAUSES

The immune system is the body's defense against infection. If it reacts abnormally and mistakenly recognizes a non-toxic substance as an invader, the white blood cells overreact causing chaos in the body.

Food dyes and binders in medications can cause allergic reactions.

Perfumes.

Mattresses, pillows and bedding are primary sources of dust allergy.

CONVENTIONAL TREATMENT

Desensitizing injections—A small amount of material causing the allergy is injected into the patient. The amount is gradually increased in the hope that antibodies will be activated to repel the foreign invader. The amount injected should not cause inflammation which comes from production of histamine from mast cells activated by the foreign matter.

Antihistamines.

Cortisone.

Decongestants.

PROBLEMS ASSOCIATED WITH CONVENTIONAL TREATMENT

Desensitizing can take up to three years before it is effective. The injections must be administered by highly experienced professionals who have the astute knowledge of determining the right quantity of the desensitizing agent. Patients given a higher amount than their body can handle can go into anaphylactic shock.

Antihistamines cause drowsiness. In fact some are even marketed as sleep aids. They also cause dryness of your mouth, nose and throat. Older men with enlarged prostate glands often have difficulty urinating when taking antihistamines.

Cortisone weakens your adrenal glands by slowing down the body's production of its own hormone. Given over long periods of time, you can form an addiction as bodily functions become dependent on it. The adrenal glands have a better opportunity to rebound if cortisone is given every other day. Additional side effects are bloating, weight gain with a moon-face appearance, retinal problems and cataracts. Cortisone also stops the absorption of protein, curtails production of male and female hormones, can cause hair growth in undesirable places in woman and breast enlargement in males. Since it is a steroid, it suppresses the immune system and makes the body more susceptible to infections. Prolonged use can also lead to psychotic behavior.

Decongestants can cause tachycardia (rapid heart beat).

ALTERNATIVE NATURAL REMEDIES

Diet

It is very important that your food be broken down into its tiniest molecule because when it is not digested properly, it can become identified as a foreign object by your immune system, which then tries to defend your body against it. Therefore, taking digestive enzymes with meals can often make a dramatic difference if you're allergic.

The most common food allergens are eggs, wheat, white potato, carrots, turnips, zucchini, avocados, runner beans, parsnips, rutabagas, milk and oranges. The three fish causing the most allergic reactions are cod, trout and plaice. In order to learn if you are allergic to a specific food, stop eating it for four days. Take your pulse, and then eat that food by itself. Wait 20 minutes and check the pulse again. If it goes up or down 10 points, a food allergy may be present.

If a person's system is too alkaline, calcium will not be broken down into an absorbable form. This interferes with cell production of histamine. Normal amounts of histamine are not harmful. It is the overproduction that causes allergic reactions. Overproduction of histamine is caused by the allergen combining with the antibody on the surface of the mast cell. This activates the release of histamine from the mast cells which causes the cells to dilate and leak fluid through their walls. In order to maintain an acid state, eat more fish, poultry, meat, whole grains, eggs (if not allergic to them), tomatoes, pomegranates, plums, prunes, nuts and seeds.

Raw honey is full of pollen and can produce a natural desensitization to many pollens.

Supplements

Vitamin D, 1000 I.U. daily for calcium absorption.

Production of histamine can be diminished by taking:

Vitamin C, 500 mg. four times daily.

Vitamin B6, 250 mg. twice daily (Always take full B complex when taking high doses of any singular B vitamin).

Bioflavanoids (quercetin), 500 mg. three times daily.

Vitamin E, 400 I.U. two times daily. (Build up to this dosage slowly as Vitamin E sometimes has a tendency to raise blood pressure.)

To stimulate the adrenal glands to produce the body's own cortisone take:

Pantothene, 500 mg. twice daily.

Herbs

Blessed thistle loosens mucous.

Pleurisy herb loosens mucous.

Black cohash relieves spasms.

Skullcap calms nerves.

Amino Acids

L-Histadine, 500 mg. twice daily, reduces the tendency to allergies by reducing the release of histamine.

Additional Information

Schizophrenics may be allergic to a particular food in one personality and a different food in another personality.

Women can be allergic to their partner's sperm.

Adhesive on postage stamps contains corn syrup, a substance causing allergic reactions in many individuals.

People who are allergic to eggs should not receive flu vaccine.

Toast bread to make it less allergic.

Anemia

DEFINITION

Anemia is a disorder marked by a deficiency in the production of red blood cells. This reduces the amount of oxygen the blood is able to carry, resulting in a lack of energy and vitality. Other symptoms include vertigo, headache, roaring in the ears, spots before the eyes, psychotic behavior and irritability.

CAUSES

The bone marrow may be incapable of producing or generating enough red cells for normal replacement needs.

Erythropoitin, the chemical the kidneys secrete for stimulating red cell production, may be lacking.

Lead poisoning. The production of heme pigment is impaired.

Chronic inflammation and extensive cancers may inhibit production of red cells.

Bleeding from gums, ulcers, hemorrhoids or heavy menstrual periods.

Antacids decrease absorption of iron.

Lack of pancreatic enzymes and hydrochloric acid. Red blood cells are made up of nutrients such as iron, B12, folic acid and copper. In order to metabolize these nutrients from food, sufficient acid and enzymes must be present in the digestive system.

A deficiency in the intrinsic factor which is needed to break down Vitamin B12.

CONVENTIONAL TREATMENT

Iron pills—325 mg.

B12 injections.

PROBLEMS ASSOCIATED WITH CONVENTIONAL TREATMENT

Iron pills and B12 injections just treat the symptoms rather than the cause of the anemia.

Iron causes constipation in most people.

The digestive system must be in an acid state for iron to be absorbed into the blood.

Too much iron in supplemental form can damage your heart, liver, pancreas and the immune system. It is stored in the tissues of your joints and can worsen arthritis.

A factor often overlooked is that Vitamin E should not be taken with an inorganic form of iron, since it will prevent iron absorption. Take these two supplements at least eight hours apart.

ALTERNATIVE NATURAL REMEDIES

Diet
Bananas contain iron and folic acid in an easily assimilable form.

Sunflower seeds contain almost as much iron as liver does.

Crude blackstrap molasses.

Black beans.

Sesame seeds and tahini.

Peas.

Egg yolks (soft cooked or poached).

Honey is rich in copper which helps iron assimilation.

Avoid caffeine which interferes with iron absorption.

Supplements
Vitamin B12, sublingually, 500 mcg. twice daily. It is important to use the sublingual form in order to bypass the stomach and intestines. The reason is that, as a person ages, the stomach and intestines lose their ability to metabolize the B12.

Iron sulfate or iron fumerate, 50 mg. twice daily.

Copper, 2 mg.

Folic Acid, 5 mg.

Manganese, 50 mg. twice a day. Manganese converts to iron in the body.

Vitamin C, 500 mg. four times a day, enhances iron absorption.

Dessicated liver powder from organic beef, 1/2 tsp. in 6 ounces of carrot juice.

Digestive enzymes such as Betaine HCL, Papain, Pepsin, Pancreatin or Bromelain—one tablet with meals. Do not take digestive enzymes if an ulcer is present.

Herbs
Red beet.

Red raspberry.

Dandelion.

Alfalfa.

All herbs ending in "dock" are high in organic iron, such as burdock and yellow dock.

Amino Acids

L-Glutathione, 500 mg. twice daily on empty stomach, aids tripeptide production of red blood cells.

L-Glycine, 500 mg. twice daily on empty stomach, is a carrier for copper, an intricate part of red blood cells.

L-Cysteine, 500 mg. once daily on empty stomach, for formation of red blood cells.

Angina

DEFINITION

Angina pectoris is a disease characterized by episodes of acute pain in the chest often accompanied with a sense of suffocation. An insufficient amount of oxygen reaches the heart muscle, leading to spasms which prevent the heart from pumping the life-sustaining blood needed in all body tissues.

CAUSES

Plaque formation thickens the coronary arteries, lowering blood flow to the heart muscle.

Inability of the heart muscle to sustain the pumping action needed to produce enough blood flow to the rest of the body.

If the heart muscle is weakened, excessive physical activity can cause an overload on it, leading to spasms causing pain.

Thickened blood, caused by fat in the diet, sugar, cholesterol, triglycerides, medications or an abnormal platelet count (clotting factor), causes a weakened heart to overexert itself in order to expel blood and pump it into the body.

"Y" shaped junctions of blood vessels, as opposed to straight, tend to pick up more debris.

Overproduction of insulin encourages growth of endothelium cells that line the blood vessels causing atherosclerosis. Too much insulin stimulates the sympathetic nervous system, leading to an increased heart rate and sodium retention, the cause of edema and bloating.

CONVENTIONAL TREATMENT

Beta blockers.
Channel blockers.
Blood pressure lowering medication.
Diuretics.
Anti-inflammatory drugs such as Prednisone and Cortisone.
Muscle relaxants.

PROBLEMS ASSOCIATED WITH CONVENTIONAL TREATMENT

Beta blockers lessen the amount of adrenalin reaching the heart muscle. This could cause a heart attack.

Channel blockers slow down the amount of calcium that reaches the heart. This may cause excessive contractions.

Blood pressure lowering medications often cause lethargy, fatigue, gout, depression and lowered thyroid metabolism.

Blood thinners thin your blood to such a degree that it is in an altered state and is unable to nourish bodily tissues with the normal amount of nutrients.

Diuretics raise insulin levels and change electrolyte balance, causing depletion of important minerals such as potassium, magnesium, calcium and chloride. They also raise uric acid levels which could lead to gout.

Prednisone and cortisone cause fluid retention and lead to weight gain, osteoporosis, inefficient absorption of proteins, swollen legs and retinal problems. Fluid retention also causes cells of the heart to enlarge and interferes with the chemical energy that is produced in the heart cell.

Muscle relaxants cause the body to lose control and strength while a person is pursuing normal daily physical activities.

ALTERNATIVE NATURAL REMEDIES

Diet And Exercise

Once a day do some form of physical exercise that does not stress the body, such as walking, swimming or light calisthenics.

Maintain normal weight and avoid the following:

Processed food.
Junk food.
Sugars.
Highly saturated fats.
Alcohol.
Smoking.

The best diet for those with any heart condition consists of:

Complex carbohydrates—fruit, fruit juices, whole wheat bread, whole wheat pasta and spaghetti, potatoes, yams, carrots, beets, brown rice, corn, beans, greens and green leafy vegetables.

High protein foods—fish, chicken, turkey, lamb, veal, non-fat cottage cheese and yogurt, low fat swiss cheese and soft cooked or poached eggs. (Never fry or scramble eggs since high heat destroys lecithin which counteracts the cholesterol in the yolk and also causes overoxidation of the fat, forming free radicals.)

Supplements

Use the following natural blood thinners, which thin the blood naturally, but only to the degree that the body needs to sustain itself, rather than lowering it so much that damage is caused.

Vitamin C, 1000 mg. four times a day.

Fish oil capsules, 300 mg. of EPA in each, 6 a day.

Lecithin, 19 gr. capsules (1200 mg.), 6 a day or 2 heaping tbsp of granules.

Evening primrose oil, 6 capsules a day.

Niacin, a natural vasodilator, 500 mg. twice a day (may cause flushing).

Garlic, enteric coated, 2000 mg. daily.

Drink at least 8 to 10 glasses of water (preferably distilled) daily. Water thins the blood naturally.

Take the following supplements also:

CoEnzyme Q10, 30 mg. three times a day, lowers blood pressure, strengthens your immune system, repairs damage from gum disease and strengthens your heart muscle.

Magnesium, potassium, bromelain combination, four a day. Magnesium is a muscle relaxant. Potassium balances the cells' pumping action with sodium. Bromelain is a natural anti-inflammatory if taken between meals.

Dimethyl glycine, 125 mg. twice daily. This is an oxygen facilitator. It allows more oxygen from your blood supply to reach your muscle and tissue cells. (The Russians used it with great success in the previous Olympics.)

Germanium, 100 mg. three a day—also an oxygen facilitator.

Herbs

Hawthorne, in tea or capsule form, per label, strengthens the heart muscle.

Amino Acids

L-Taurine, 500 mg. four times daily on empty stomach, is a natural diuretic, moderates cholesterol production and prevents cardiac loss of potassium.

L-Carnitine, 500 mg. twice daily, burns excess fat in the heart muscle cells as energy. It is also effective for weight loss.

L-Glutamine, 500 mg. four times daily, reduces the loss of potassium and sodium electrolytes.

L-Histadine, 500 mg. twice daily, widens your arteries.

Anorexia Nervosa

DEFINITION

Anorexia Nervosa is an undereating disorder occurring primarily in adolescents and young teenage females. Those who suffer from this condition are obsessed with the idea that they are fat. In order to keep up appearances, they will partake of food. Afterward, manifesting a related disease, Bulimia, many force themselves to regurgitate in order to rid themselves of food, which they regard as an enemy.

CAUSES

Severe zinc deficiency which can affect the taste buds.

Psychological factors. These young females think they will not be accepted socially if they are overweight. Though they may be sylph-like when they observe their reflection in the mirror, they see a fat person. The problem often begins with parents who require too much from a child who does not have the capacity to conform to these demands. Some self-starve themselves to the point of death from malnutrition.

CONVENTIONAL TREATMENT

Psychological therapy/psychological medicine.

PROBLEMS ASSOCIATED WITH CONVENTIONAL TREATMENT

Psychological therapy usually fails because therapists are treating a problem that should have been addressed before it began. However, our society frowns upon preventive programs. A more successful type of therapy would be to strengthen the patient's self-esteem and self-love so that extraneous circumstances would not have such a great effect.

Many of these patients have problems with their taste buds, a factor often overlooked by orthodox medical practitioners.

ALTERNATIVE NATURAL REMEDIES

Diet

A strict diet consisting of natural organic type food should be provided in place of standard American fare of processed foods, sugar, fast foods, alcohol, junk food and highly overcooked restaurant foods. Frequent small meals may be more easily tolerated.

Supplements

Multi-vitamin and mineral combination such as VM75.

Zinc picolinate, 50 mg. twice daily. This can give dramatic results with anorexia since a zinc deficiency can cause the taste buds to malfunction to the degree that food loses all its flavor.

Herbs

The following herbs all enhance the appetite:

Saw palmetto berries.

Horseradish.

Hops.

Mustard.

Caraway.

Alfalfa.

Folic Acid.

Philotherapy (Philosophy Therapy)

The therapist must be able to convince the patient that being overly thin is not a desirable quality. It is important to find a therapist who has the ability to understand how anorexics perceive themselves. When these patients decide that the information they are receiving from the therapist is believable, they begin to change how they perceive themselves.

Parents attempt to strengthen their own egos by absorbing the accomplishments of their children. The children may be inadequate and unable to accomplish the goals set by the parents. This forces the child to overcompensate for what he or she cannot do. Eventually the stress and pressures lead to the psychological manifestation of anorexia.

ARTHRITIS

DEFINITION

Although arthritis can take many different forms, the two most common are rheumatoid arthritis and osteoarthritis.

Rheumatoid arthritis is a disease of the autoimmune system which overreacts to foreign matter in the joints. This overreaction causes deterioration of the synovial membranes surrounding lubricating fluid in the joints. Bone and cartilage are damaged, and the body replaces the degenerated areas with scar tissue, thereby narrowing the spaces between the joints.

Osteoarthritis is an age related disease caused by continual friction between bones. This initiates an inflammatory process leading to stiffness and pain. Osteoarthritis can also be the result of high intensity exercise and sports.

CAUSES

Rheumatoid Arthritis

Genetics—An individual may be predisposed to a genetic dysfunction of the immune system.

Dietary—Certain foods, such as those in the nightshade family including white potatoes, eggplant, green peppers, tomatoes and tobacco contain the toxin, solanaise, that causes inflammation in the joints.

Both children and adults exhibiting symptoms of rheumatoid arthritis should be checked for Lyme's Disease.

Osteoarthritis

Physical activity—Constant use of the same muscle causes breakdown of the structure's supporting fibers. This causes weakness in the area and eventually leads to pain, stiffness and disability.

Nutritional—A deficiency in the nutrients that form collagen tissue (the material that holds the body together). The support system of the body fails, causing pressure on weakened joints which then become inflamed.

When inflammation occurs, blood vessels invade the cartilage and break it up. This is similar to what happens when water gets into a crack in concrete and freezes, causing it to crack.

Deficiencies in the nutrients that feed muscles, ligaments and tendons will prevent them from operating in the manner of their design.

Fluorine added to the water supply to strengthen teeth and bones, also causes unneeded bone growth in arthritic joints.

CONVENTIONAL TREATMENT

Surgery for replacement of the diseased joint.

Physical therapy, including specific exercises, heat treatments, steam baths, swimming and whirlpool baths.

Medications, including cortisone, non-steroid anti-inflammatory drugs and muscle relaxants.

Gold Therapy.

Devices such as back and knee braces, elastic bandages and cervical collars.

PROBLEMS ASSOCIATED WITH CONVENTIONAL TREATMENT

Surgery requires a long hospital stay, is expensive and has a high failure rate, especially for back operations. It treats only the symptoms without addressing the true cause of the disability. Scar tissue attracts bacteria and fungi to the area. The bacteria and fungi then attack the tissue, causing it to become inflamed and leading to further deterioration. Some patients are hypersensitive to the nickel used in hip replacements.

Physical therapy, although effective, is expensive and time consuming and requires a high degree of commitment on the part of the patient. Swimming pools have a six inch blanket of chlorine which settles on top of the water. As swimmers exert energy, they inhale large amounts of chlorine which is meant to destroy bacteria. The problem is that chlorine also destroys the body's friendly bacteria. This leaves the body vulnerable to attack by disease-carrying bacteria and viruses. Swimmers should seek unpolluted open water or use pools purified with bromine.

Medications all have side effects. Cortisone weakens your adrenal glands by slowing down the body's production of its own hormone. Given over long periods of time, you can form an addiction as bodily functions become dependent on it. The adrenal glands have a better opportunity to rebound if cortisone is given every other day. Other side effects are bloating, weight gain with a moon-face appearance, retinal problems and cataracts. Cortisone also stops the absorption of protein and curtails production of male and female hormones. It can also cause hair growth in undesirable places in women and breast enlargement in men. Since it is a steroid, it suppresses the immune system and makes the body more susceptible to infections. Prolonged use can also lead to psychotic behavior.

Non-steroid anti-inflammatories can cause dizziness, nausea, headache, constipation, diarrhea and vomiting.

Muscle relaxants may cause lethargy, weakness, sleepiness, difficulty urinating, rapid heart beat, unsteadiness and a bad taste in the mouth. After a period of nine to ten months, patients require higher dosages of these medications in order for them to be effective.

Gold therapy takes a long time to be effective. Benefits derived are not equal to the side effects, time and cost of the treatment. In addition, heavy metals poison the system and cause disruption of cell metabolism.

Devices that restrict motion can cause joints to atrophy from lack of use.

ALTERNATIVE NATURAL REMEDIES

Arthritis is caused when your system becomes too alkaline. Calcium should be made soluble by the body and be transported into the proper cells. Instead, calcium accumulates in your joints and tissues and causes bursitis, tendonitis, heel spurs and osteoarthritis. This high alkaline state can be corrected by changing your body to an acid state.

Diet

Foods that activate an acid state are:

Grains, except millet and buckwheat.

Nuts, except almonds and Brazil nuts.

Natural cheese.

Lentils.

Animal protein such as meat, fish and poultry, organic only.

Cider vinegar, 2 tsp. in a glass of low sodium vegetable juice twice a day.

Avoid foods in the nightshade family since they contain solinaise, which inflames the synovial fluid in the joints.

Supplements

Geri-Vital for pain relief.

Shark cartilage (Cartilade), as directed on label, reduces the inflammatory process and prevents the blood vessels from invading the cartilage of your joints.

Bromelain, 500 mg. twice a day.

Omega 3 (fish oil), 1000 mg. EPA twice a day (6 capsules).

Sea cucumber (Seacare) as directed on label.

Vitamin C, 1000 mg. three times a day, to rebuild collagen and make the body more acid.

Pantothene, 500 mg. twice daily, acts as an anti-inflammatory.

Herbs

Yucca helps to stimulate the adrenal glands to produce the body's own cortisone.

Black cohosh relieves pain and inflammation.

Hydrangea acts like cortisone, but without the cost or side effects.

Alfalfa increases vitality.

Amino Acids

L-Proline, per label, helps rebuild deteriorating joint linings.

L-Cysteine, 500 mg. twice daily on empty stomach, is essential for immune function.

L-Lysine, 500 mg. three times daily on empty stomach, reduces the inflammatory response of antibodies.

Adjunctive Procedures

Castor oil packs. Soak a piece of white flannel in warm castor oil, wring it out and place over the inflamed area. Cover with plastic and apply a heating pad. Do this twice a day for one hour each sitting.

Acupuncture, acupressure and massage open energy pathways on meridians leading to the organs that produce the body's own healing power and stimulate the body's lymph system which cleanses the blood of toxins.

T.E.N.S. (transcutaneous electrical nerve stimulation) unit to help with pain.

Mexitil, a prescription drug, is excellent for pain relief, and has the least amount of side effects.

Trigger point colchicine for pain.

Cobra venom injections (given by holistic medical doctor) reduce inflammation.

Zostrex cream (capsicum-cayenne red pepper extract) soothes inflamed joints.

ASTHMA

DEFINITION

Asthma is a respiratory disorder characterized by difficulty in breathing. Following association with allergic material, the airways contract, allowing less oxygen in and less carbon dioxide out of the body. The allergic reaction also produces fluid and swelling of the airways.

CAUSES

Allergy to irritants such as dust, dander, molds, smog, dust mites and industrial pollutants.

Cold temperatures can contract the airways.

Strenuous exercise.

Emotional factors can cause depression of the immune system leading to an autoimmune attack to the lungs.

Nasal polyps, caused by an alkaline state.

IgG subclass deficiency (rare).

CONVENTIONAL TREATMENT

Cortisone.

Bronchodilators, in oral or aerosol form.

Muscle relaxants.

Relocation to areas with dry climate such as Arizona.

PROBLEMS ASSOCIATED WITH CONVENTIONAL TREATMENT

Cortisone weakens the adrenal glands by slowing down the body's production of its own hormone. Given over long periods of time, the patient can form an addiction as bodily functions become dependent on it. The adrenal glands have a better opportunity to rebound if cortisone is given every other day. Other side effects are bloating, weight gain with a moon-face appearance, retinal problems and cataracts. Cortisone also stops the absorption of protein, curtails production of male and female hormones, can cause hair growth in undesirable places in women and breast enlargement in males. Women's voices may become deeper. Since it is a steroid, it suppresses the immune system and makes the body more susceptible to infections. Prolonged use can also lead to psychotic behavior.

Bronchodilators can cause lethargy and can begin to shut off your own respiratory system. You become overly dependent on the drugs, and do not heal on your own as well. These drugs may also cause blood pressure changes and/or tachycardia.

Muscle relaxants can cause lethargy, weakness, sleepiness, difficulty in urinating, rapid heart beat, unsteadiness and a bad taste in the mouth.

Relocation is expensive, often impractical, and it is stressful to leave one's family, friends and roots.

ALTERNATIVE NATURAL REMEDIES

If a severe asthmatic attack occurs and no medication is available, drink a cup of strong coffee or place a slice of onion under your tongue. These act as bronchodilators. Theopheline, a bronchodilator, is one of the main constituents of caffeine.

Diet

Asthmatics have low blood sugar. Diabetics, with their high blood sugar, seldom have asthma. Normalize blood sugar levels by avoiding high carbohydrates, sugars and highly processed foods. An exception is raw, certified, locally processed honey, which helps build immunity by acting as a barrier against inhaled pollens. Start with small amounts.

Avoid wheat products, canned foods, dairy products, sugar, and salt. Citrus fruits can cause an allergic effect unless they are tree-ripened. Asthmatics should be tested for food allergies and avoid all foods that cause reactions. Some chiropractors are now testing for food allergies by using a muscle kinesiology system. This is non-invasive, accurate and inexpensive. Other tests for food allergies are scratch tests, RAST blood test and cytotoxic blood testing.

Cayenne pepper, hot peppers, coffee, horseradish and mustard all act as vasodilators. (A word of caution—all may raise blood pressure).

Honey clears the lungs and soothes coughing spasms.

Grape juice clears mucous and phlegm from the lungs.

Sour fruits such as pineapple and berries help dissolve mucous.

Barley water contains hordenine, which relieves bronchial spasms.

Raw onion acts as an expectorant. It is so potent that bronchial spasms can often be relieved by simply sucking on a slice of onion.

Supplements

Vitamin B6, 250 mg. three times daily, acts as an antihistamine. Check with a nutritional medical doctor periodically as this is a high dosage.

Magnesium citrate or magnesium aspartate, 500 mg. three times daily, acts as a muscle relaxant. Cut back on dosage if diarrhea occurs.

Vitamin C, 1000 mg. three times daily, acts as an antihistamine.

Quercetin (Bioflavanoids), 500 mg. four times daily, acts as an antihistamine and also stabilizes the membrane of the cell, enabling it to repel the offending allergen.

Vitamin A (from fish liver oil), 25,000 I.U. once daily.

Vitamin A (Beta carotene), 25,000 I.U. once daily.

Bee pollen, either capsules or in granular form. Start with small amount and gradually build up. The effect is similar to desensitization against the patient's allergen if it is to pollen from plants such as ragweed, golden rod, etc.

Myers Cocktail. This is an intravenous procedure administered by holistic physicians. It contains Vitamin C, Vitamin B12, Vitamin B6, magnesium, calcium and folic acid.

Herbs

Blessed thistle strengthens your lungs and loosens mucous and phlegm.

Pleurisy herb loosens mucous.

Golden seal reduces swelling.

Marshmallow herb (not the confection) relaxes your bronchial tubes.

Lobelia acts as an expectorant and relieves spasms.

Mullein is an expectorant.

Amino Acid

L-Methionine, 500 mg. twice daily on empty stomach, is an anti-oxidant.

Breathing Exercises

The average person uses less than 60 percent of lung capacity because of improper breathing. Yoga type breathing is highly recommended. Include some type of mild aerobic exercise such as walking, swimming in non-chlorinated water, cycling or light calisthenics. Avoid strenuous exercise and contact sports since they can induce asthmatic attacks.

BACK PROBLEMS

DEFINITION

Mild to severe pain and aching, usually in the lower back, often accompanied by muscle spasms and immobilization.

CAUSES

Osteoarthritis.

Injuries and accidents.

Degeneration of the joints, ligaments, muscles or intervertebral discs.

Heavy lifting.

Inactivity.

Structural defects such as swayback, scoliosis, difference in leg length.

Poor posture.

Sports involving twisting, lifting, bending, sudden starts and stops and jumping.

Exercising before muscles are warmed up.

Getting up from bed or a seated position in the wrong way.

CONVENTIONAL TREATMENT

Traction and/or bed rest.

Surgery, such as laminectomy or fusion of the spine.

Myelogram for diagnostic purposes.

Injection of the intervertebral disc with chemo papain.

Medications.

Braces.

PROBLEMS ASSOCIATED WITH CONVENTIONAL TEATMENT

Traction produces a high level of discomfort.

The inactivity of bed rest causes deterioration of your muscles, ligaments and tendons.

Back surgery has only a 50 percent success rate and even then your problem will often recur.

A myelogram is a dangerous procedure as the patient can have an adverse reaction to the dye injected into the spine.

Braces should be worn only during an acute spasmodic episode, because you can become dependent on a back brace, and it slows your healing process.

All medications have side effects.

ALTERNATIVE NATURAL REMEDIES

Prevention

Most back problems are caused by weakened muscles, ligaments and tendons which have lost their ability to support the back. Specific back-strengthening exercises can be learned under the supervision of a physical therapist or physiatrist. An emphasis should be placed on stretching the hamstrings and the abdominal muscles.

Swimming in non-chlorinated water is an excellent back exercise since the gravity force on the body is much less. Walking in waist-high water, cycling, rowing, stretching, walking and yoga are all good activities to maintain a strong supple back.

Try not to sleep on the back or stomach. The best position is on the side with the legs bent. Do not jump out of bed too fast. Sit on the edge of the bed for a few minutes first.

When sitting for long periods, try to keep the knees higher than the hips. Never arise too fast. Place hands on the knees before standing. When driving, sit as far forward as comfort allows and use a back support for the seat.

Try to avoid wearing high heels since they cause misalignment of the spine.

Diet

Avoid foods in the nightshade family, such as potatoes, tomatoes, eggplant, tobacco and peppers if the problem is caused by arthritic changes.

Animal foods and sugar cause the loss of oxygen in the bloodstream which eventually slows healing.

Supplements

DLPA (DL Phenylalanine), 500 mg. four times daily on empty stomach, releases endorphins, your body's own painkillers. This must be taken at least seven days to be effective. But you must cut down on the dosage after your pain is relieved.

Bromelain, 500 mg. twice daily, acts as an anti-inflammatory.

Pantothene, 500 mg. twice daily, acts as an anti-inflammatory.

Vitamin B1 (thiamine), 250 mg. twice daily, acts as a muscle relaxant.

Vitamin B12 sublingual, 1000 mcg. twice daily, cuts down nervous tension so your body, and especially your back, can relax.

Vitamin C, 1000 mg. three times daily, to build up the collagen that strengthens and rebuilds your back muscles. Use buffered "C" to alleviate heartburn from high dosage of "C".

Herbs

Valerian root is a relaxant.

Yucca is an anti-inflammatory.

Licorice root cleanses the liver of toxins.

Ginger aids circulation.

Amino Acids

Branch chain amino acids such as L-Leucine, L-Isoleucine and L-Valine, as directed on label, strengthen and rebuild muscles.

L-Argenine, 1000 mg. three times daily on empty stomach, helps bring energy to those weakened back muscles.

L-Phenylalanine, 500 mg. three times daily on empty stomach, elevates endorphins.

Adjunctive Remedies

Trigger point injections of colchicine, administered by physician, to relieve pain.

Acupuncture.

Acupressure.

Massage.

Reflexology treatments.

Chiropractic adjustments.

Bed board.

T.E.N.S. (transcuteneous electrical nerve stimulation) for alleviation of pain.

Castor oil packs. Dip a piece of white flannel into some warm castor oil, wring out and place over affected area. Cover with plastic and apply a heating pad for one hour. Use twice daily for one week.

BALDING

DEFINITION

Balding is the loss of some or all of the hair on the head. It may be a sign that the internal organs are becoming weak.

CAUSES

Genetics.

Overproduction of testosterone, the male sex hormone, which causes thickened galea, a sheet of tissue on top of the scalp. This results in constriction of the blood capillaries in the scalp and impaired blood supply to the hair roots. Males tend to lose elasticity in the galea, but this membrane usually remains thin and elastic in females.

Stress causes muscle tension and constriction of blood vessels in the scalp, leading to a slowdown in the circulation of blood to the hair root and follicle.

Radiation—X-Rays trigger destruction of the DNA (mastermind of the cell), cause the cell to die and bring on baldness.

Thyroid imbalance—Iodine deficiency causes the improper production of thyroxine, which is made in the thyroid.gland. When insufficient thyroxine is produced, dryness, thinness and poor hair growth occurs.

A deficiency of Vitamin F or essential fatty acids will lead to the improper secretion of sebum from the sebaceous glands. Over or underproduction of sebum can lead to an unhealthy condition of hair follicles and roots.

Vitamin A deficiency can lead to excessive dandruff and a dry, itchy, flaky scalp, which can cause weakening of the hair root and eventual loss of hair.

Constant wearing of a hat.

Overuse of shampoos or washing hair too often.

Overexposure to the sun.

CONVENTIONAL TREATMENT

Minoxidil, a drug used originally to lower blood pressure.

Over the counter hair restorers.

Hair transplants.

Hormone therapy. Estrogen, a female hormone, is given to males to balance out the overproduction of testosterone.

PROBLEMS ASSOCIATED WITH CONVENTIONAL TREATMENT

Minoxidil is very expensive. It can also cause lowering of your blood pressure as it is absorbed through the scalp into the bloodstream. In order for it to work, it must be used on an ongoing basis as hair loss will recur if the treatment is stopped.

Most over-the-counter hair restorers are not effective.

Hair transplants are painful and extremely expensive, somewhere in the $10,000 range. There is also the possibility of infection. Sometimes the procedure fails and must be repeated.

Use of the female hormone, estrogen, may have side effects in males, such as breast enlargement, a higher pitch to the voice and an increase in feminine characteristics.

ALTERNATIVE NATURAL REMEDIES

Diet

Excess salt in the diet can lead to hair loss. It causes an imbalance in the electrolytes (minerals) which are needed for proper nourishment.

Sebaceous glands are affected by high intake of refined carbohydrates and too much fat in the diet. Sugar converts to fat in the body and fat causes the glands to produce too much oil leading to clogging of the hair follicles.

Supplements

Iodine, 150 mg. daily, aids in the production of thyroxin from the thyroid gland. When insufficient thyroxine is produced from your thyroid gland, poor hair growth and thinness of your hair occurs. Iodine directly aids in your body's production of that vital thyroxin, and thus that hair growth. A diet rich in fish and sea food would be the best source of iodine, but for those who don't like fish or can't tolerate it, the best source is from the sea vegetable, kelp.

Vitamin E, 400 I.U.

Wheat germ oil, 4 capsules daily.

Beta carotene A, 50,000 I.U. daily.

Vitamin C, 500 mg. three times daily.

Biotin, 5 mg. daily—you also need Biotin because your hair follicles are made up of cysteine and biotin.

Manganese, 50 mg. twice daily.

Vitamin F (essential fatty acids), according to label.

The following three supplements also aid in maintaining or restoring hair color. Take them along with a 50 mg. B complex.

PABA, 300 mg. twice daily.

Pantothene, 300 mg. three times daily.

Folic acid, 5 mg. daily.

Herbs

Cayenne—increases circulation.

Ginger—increases circulation.

Horsetail—helps supply calcium for hair and nails.

Nettles—has been used for centuries as a hair stimulant.

Amino Acids

L-Cysteine, 500 mg. twice daily. It is important for those with a predisposition to kidney stones to take three times as much Vitamin C as cysteine (3000 mg. of Vitamin C).

Other Natural Approaches

Brushing cleans the scalp of dirt, dandruff and dead skin and helps stimulate the sebaceous glands to release their secretions.

Massage the scalp with fingers or a vibrator.

Headstands, or lying on a slant board, brings fresh blood to the area and nourishes the scalp.

BLOOD PRESSURE
(HYPERTENSION)

DEFINITION

High blood pressure is not a disease per se, rather it is the body's attempt to deal with an abnormal situation. Ideally, blood pressure should be 120/80, and can vary from 110 to 140 over 60 to 95. The upper reading is called systolic. It occurs when the heart contracts and forces blood through the circulatory system. The bottom reading is the diastolic and occurs when the heart fills with blood in its expansion phase and the blood pressure is at its lowest. This is also known as the resting state. The diastolic is the more important reading since the heart and the arteries are in the expansion phase 75 percent of the time. If diastolic pressure is elevated, there is more stress on the arteries and the heart.

It is ineffective to continually treat the symptom of high blood pressure without addressing the cause.

CAUSES

Obesity.

Emotional factors.

Kidney problems.

High sodium intake.

High sugar intake.

General toxic condition.

Medicines.

Arteriosclerosis (hardening of the arteries) puts more effort on the heart.

Atherosclerosis (narrowing of the arteries) puts more effort on the heart.

Imbalance of electrolytes (calcium, magnesium, sodium, potassium).

Imbalanced endocrine system, malfunctioning of adrenal glands.

High cholesterol.

Smoking constricts all arteries and capillaries, causing the heart to pump harder to force blood through them.

Alcohol consumption destroys liver cells which produce chemicals in the body needed for healthy living.

CONVENTIONAL TREATMENT

Diuretics.

Beta Blockers.

Calcium channel blockers.

Diet and weight loss.

Salt restriction.

Vasodilator drugs.

PROBLEMS ASSOCIATED WITH CONVENTIONAL TREATMENT

All drugs have undesirable side effects. Drugs used for high blood pressure often cause all of the following: depression, fatigue, sexual problems, loss of appetite and electrolyte imbalance. If blood pressure is lowered too much, dizziness can occur, leading to falls and broken bones. Other drugs, whether prescription or over-the-counter, can interact with blood pressure medication, causing dangerous adverse effects, and some foods such as aged cheese, herring, etc. can also have bad effects with certain medications.

Patients on diuretics also excrete trace minerals, the lack of which may be a cause of Altzheimers disease. Potassium depletion from diuretics impairs insulin release. Diuretics also raise cholesterol. They lower excretion of uric acid which builds up in the joints, possibly causing gout.

ALTERNATIVE NATURAL REMEDIES

Diet

Cucumbers, onions, garlic and watermelon act as natural diuretics.

Bananas contain mono amines, a chemical compound that raises blood pressure. People on diuretics are told to eat bananas to replace lost potassium, yet they are actually raising their blood pressure.

Supplements

Vitamin C (Ester C), 1000 mg. three times daily, acts as a diuretic and helps clear your arteries of plaque.

Vitamin B6, 100 mg. three times daily, acts as a diuretic.

B complex, 50 mg. twice daily, for calming of nerves.

Fish oil (EPA), 1000 mg. twice daily, lowers blood pressure.

Niacin, 250 mg. twice daily, acts as a vasodilator, opening arteries and alleviating high blood pressure by allowing more efficient blood flow. Be aware of niacin flush, a feeling of heat and flushing in upper torso, arms and face. Cut back on dosage if this occurs. Do not use time-release niacin because it can have a deleterious effect on the liver.

Magnesium citrate, 500 mg. twice daily, acts as a muscle relaxant and overall antispasmodic.

Calcium citrate, 500 mg., is effective as a stress reducer and relaxant, especially if taken before bed. If calcium and magnesium are taken in a combined form, be sure the ratio is two parts magnesium to one part calcium.

Potassium, 500 mg. twice daily.

Vitamin E reduces blood pressure if taken in small amounts initially. Start with 100 I.U. daily and gradually raise the dosage biweekly until taking 600 I.U. daily.

Herbs

Hawthorn strengthens the heart muscle.

Cayenne red pepper for circulation.

Garlic opens up blood vessels.

Parsley is a natural diuretic.

Juniper berries act as a diuretic.

Uva ursi acts as a diuretic.

Buchu acts as a diuretic.

Marshmallow root strengthens the kidneys.

Amino Acids

L-Taurine, 500 mg. four times daily on empty stomach, reduces loss of potassium and acts as a natural diuretic.

L-Tryptophan, 500 mg. three times daily (from pure sources) on empty stomach, is a calming neurotransmitter.

L-Valine, 500 mg. four times daily on empty stomach, promotes restful sleep, stabilizes emotions and nervousness.

L-Glutamine, 500 mg. four times daily on empty stomach, reduces potassium and sodium electrolyte loss.

L-Isoleucine, per label, reduces stress to the central nervous system.

Stress Reduction

Individuals must change their interpretation and perception of extraneous events. A negative perception causes anxiety and/or depression, which in turn increases adrenalin production leading to an increase in blood pressure.

This can be accomplished by raising self-esteem to such a degree that outside influences do not affect a person's psychological well-being. Patients must learn how to control themselves in situations that have a negative influence on them by means of meditation, biofeedback, affirmations, self-discipline, control and commitment. Then they will be in charge of the situation instead of being controlled by the whims of the economic and sociological demands of society.

An optimistic viewpoint must be maintained at all times. It has been shown that optimism raises the immune system to such a high degree that it counteracts the negative effects of any illness.

BOWEL PROBLEMS (COLON)

DEFINITION

A well functioning colon should store and evacuate fecal matter easily. The colon also reabsorbs fluids. Problems occur when the colon becomes inflamed or when waste material moves too slowly (constipation) or too rapidly (diarrhea) through the large bowel. Yeast overgrowth (Candida albicans) can occur from the proliferation of too many negative bacteria and cause inflammatory conditions.

CAUSES

Diverticulitis.

Colitis.

Crohn's Disease.

Irritable bowel syndrome.

Colon cancer.

Appendicitis.

Polyps.

Tumors.

Food allergies.

Parasites.

Undigested proteins. (Indicin urine test should be utilized to see if this condition exists).

Low back problems should be investigated as a possible cause of colon malfunctions.

CONVENTIONAL TREATMENT

Anti-inflammatory drugs such as cortisone.

Asulfidine.

Surgical procedures.

Chemotherapy and radiation.

Dietary changes to high fiber or to low residue.

Laxative type medications.

PROBLEMS ASSOCIATED WITH CONVENTIONAL TREATMENT

Cortisone weakens the adrenal glands by slowing down the body's production of its own hormone. Given over long periods of time, the patient can form an addiction as bodily functions become dependent on it. The adrenal glands have a better opportunity to rebound if cortisone is given every other day. Additional side effects are bloating, weight gain with a moon-face appearance, retinal problems and cataracts. Cortisone also stops the absorption of protein, curtails production of male and female hormones, can cause hair growth in undesirable places in woman and breast enlargement in males. Since it is a steroid, it suppresses the immune system and makes the body more susceptible to infections. Prolonged use can also lead to psychotic behavior.

Asulfidine can cause itching or a skin rash, sensitivity to the sun, loss of appetite, aching and weakness. It depletes the body of folic acid which is needed to suppress inflammatory conditions of the bowels.

Surgical procedures treat the symptomatic problems and do not address the underlying condition. They also cause scar tissue and adhesions to form, the results of which can be a worse problem than the original condition.

The side effects of chemotherapy are so horrendous to many individuals that they discontinue treatment and turn to another modality. Chemotherapy not only destroys the virus, but also kills or weakens existing cells and the immune system. Other side effects are peeling skin, sores in the mouth, nausea and hair loss.

Radiation causes death to the DNA in cells of the area being irradiated. The function of other organs and glands in the area is impaired or compromised.

Laxatives become addictive to the point that a normal bowel movement can no longer take place without their stimulation since the colon loses the ability to operate on its own.

A low residue diet slows down the entire digestive system, interferes with its normal function and may cause constipation in certain individuals. However, it may have to be employed if there is a high degree of inflammation.

A diagnostic method, colonoscopy, can loosen bacteria. The bacteria can then collect on the mitral valve of the heart, leading to endocarditis or rheumatic fever.

ALTERNATIVE NATURAL REMEDIES
Diet
Cabbage juice and potato juice help replenish the normal flora and enhance healing.

High fiber diet such as bran, fruits with skin, brown rice, whole grain breads and pasta.

Green leafy vegetables for cellulose.

Papaya aids digestion.

Figs, prunes, and dates are natural laxatives.

Yogurt with active cultures replenishes friendly bacteria.

Buttermilk produces friendly bacteria in the colon.

Water, preferably spring or distilled, eight to ten glasses a day to soften stools.

Fasting eliminates inflammation and helps heal tissue. Fast for three days, taking only water, fruit and vegetable juices.

Apple cider vinegar, 2 tsp. in a glass of vegetable juice, acts as a digestive enzyme. Do not use if stomach ulcers are present.

Avoid processed food, junk food, fast food, fried food, chemicals and additives, artificial food coloring, foods with a high sugar content, alcohol, spices and nuts and seeds.

Supplements
Vitamin A Beta carotene, 25,000 I.U. four times daily, helps keep cavities in intestine, resulting from colitis, from growing larger. These cavities absorb undigested food, bacteria and impurities which then enter the bloodstream, causing toxic reactions.

Folic acid, 40 to 60 mg. daily, helps replace the folic acid that is lost by the action of asulfadine. Folic acid also stimulates the production of hydrochloric acid which helps prevent parasites and food poisoning. This strength can be obtained only with a prescription since high doses of folic acid can mask pernicious anemia.

Pantothene, 300 mg. three times daily, acts as an anti-inflammatory.

Acidophilus, enteric coated, 2 billion viable cells each, four times daily, to restore your intestinal flora.

Digestive enzymes in combination form to break food particles into their tiniest parts and enable digestion to take place in the proper part of your intestinal tract. When food particles are not assimilated properly before they arrive in the colon, they can act as an allergen.

Aloe vera gel, 2 ounces three times daily. This is extremely important for healing irritated and inflamed intestinal tissues. (Store aloe vera gel in the refrigerator).

Herbs

Comfrey soothes, heals and strengthens tissues.

Marshmallow root contains mucilage which helps in healing.

Ginger relieves gas and settles stomach.

Lobelia removes obstructions of mucous.

Peppermint oil aids digestion.

Slippery elm acts as an anti-inflammatory.

Cascara, sagrada and senna are natural laxatives.

Psyllium seed husks are bulking agents.

Swill Kress as a laxative.

Super Dieters Tea by Lacey Le Beau as a laxative.

Amino Acids

L-Histadine, 500 mg. twice daily on empty stomach, helps promote stomach digestive secretions, aiding in the breakdown of food particles which, if not digested, can cause inflammation in the bowel.

L-Taurine, 500 mg. three times daily on empty stomach, is a precursor of bile, aiding in the digestion of fats which, if not digested properly, can cause inflammatory bowel problems.

Adjunctive Remedies

Colonics administered by colonic therapist.

Coffee enemas help release imbedded toxins in wall of your colon and also stimulate liver to release toxins from the entire system, thereby providing a healthy body state. To prepare, perk two tablespoons of coffee in one quart of distilled water. Cool to body temperature. Take one pint and retain for ten minutes. Expel and repeat with the second pint. A special bag and tube can be ordered from Mr. David Sauder 1-800-999-2700. Patients with colostomies should not use coffee enemas.

Castor oil packs placed over the lower abdomen alleviate pain and inflammation and aid healing. To prepare, soak a piece of white flannel in warm castor oil. Place on affected area, cover with plastic and apply a heating pad for one to one and a half hours.

Breast Disease
(FIBROCYSTIC)

DEFINITION

Benign fluid-filled cysts surrounded by fibrous tissue may be firm or soft and usually move freely. These cysts are most often tender and change in size during the menstrual cycle (hormonally related). Soft lumps are usually not malignant. Hard lumps have more of a tendency to be malignant. All breast lumps should be evaluated by a physician.

CAUSES

The orthodoxy has not determined the cause of fibrocystic breast disease other than to relate it to a disturbance of cyclic breast changes taking place during the menstrual cycle. Holistic or natural healing physicians have arrived at the following determinants.

Accumulation and overproduction of toxins which cause the destruction of the DNA of the cell.

Underactive thyroid, which slows body metabolism and deactivates the normal growing process of the cell, causing it to take on an increased amount of fluid and enlarge.

Overproduction of the active form of estrogen which appears in the female body at the ovulatory phase.

A possible side effect of caffeine.

CONVENTIONAL TREATMENT

Needle aspiration to withdraw fluid.

Surgical removal of the cyst.

Antihormonal drugs.

Periodic observation by mammography.

PROBLEMS ASOCIATED WITH CONVENTIONAL TREATMENT

Aspiration does not affect the underlying problem. The fluid may return.

Side effects of surgery are pain and scarring.

Antihormonal drugs disrupt other hormones in the body such as prolactin and progesterone, which may lead to further imbalance, and possible uterine bleeding. Since these drugs are synthetic rather than natural hormones, they do not work in the same manner in the body and may lead to atrophy of other hormone producing glands.

Mammography is an X-ray and may cause destruction of the DNA in the cell which may eventually may lead to the beginning of a malignant tumor. The benefits of early detection of cancer may outweigh the risks. Be sure the doctor's equipment is dedicated (used only for mammograms), has been manufactured after 1987 and does not deliver more than a total of 200 millirads for the study—50 millirads per view, two views each breast. How do you find out this information? Ask. If you do not get a satisfactory answer, have the mammogram done elsewhere.

ALTERNATIVE NATURAL REMEDIES

Diet

Eliminate all animal foods with the exception of low fat fish and non-fat dairy products such as yogurt and non-fat cottage cheese. The reason is that animals have been given hormones which are fat-soluble elements that accumulate in their tissues and milk.

Avoid caffeine which is in coffee, chocolate, cola and tea, except certain herbal teas. Be aware that many sodas other than colas also contain caffeine.

No fried food, processed food, junk food or sugar.

The diet should consist of complex carbohydrates, including fruit, greens, whole grains, beans, starchy vegetables, nuts and seeds. Although nuts and seeds contain some fat, it is of a different composition and not derived from man-altered animals.

Supplements

Vitamin E, 800 I.U., to thin the blood (work up to this dose slowly).

Vitamin C, 500 mg. four times daily, acts as an antioxidant to protect the D.N.A. of your breast cells.

Vitamin A (Beta carotene), 25,000 I.U. twice daily, protects benign cysts from becoming malignant.

Lipotropic factors (inositol, choline and methionine), 2000 mg. daily.

Iodine, 150 mcg. twice daily, to enhance the thyroid. The best form is from the sea vegetable, kelp. Iodine aids in the development and functioning of the thyroid gland and is an integral part of thyroxine, a principal hormone produced by the gland, which regulates metabolism.

A good multi-vitamin/mineral supplement such as VM75.

Herbs

Licorice root has the same effect as antihormone drugs on the receptor sites of breast cells. It blocks these receptor sites and prevents active estrogen from proliferating.

Chaparral cleans your breasts of toxic waste.

Yellow dock nourishes the liver and spleen.

Red clover eliminates toxins.

Sarsaparilla increases the metabolic rate.

Detox tea.

GLA in the form of borage oil 240, twice daily.

Amino Acids

L-Glutathione, 500 mg. twice daily on empty stomach, is an immune stimulant and detoxifies free radicals.

L-Methionine, 500 mg. twice daily on empty stomach, reduces estrogen to estradiol, a less active form. It also prevents fat cohesion in the liver, allowing it to deactivate overactive estrogen.

Adjunctive Remedies

Apply vitamin E oil topically twice daily over the area of the cyst.

Castor oil rubbed in twice daily alleviates pain and inflammation.

An excellent product for hormonal balance is Progestade. It is applied to the skin and eventually absorbed into the bloodstream. It is not available in stores but can be ordered by calling 1-800-648-8211 or by writing to Box 3427, Eugene, Oregon 97403.

By following these recommendations, existing cysts may disappear and the initiation process of new cysts may not occur.

These recommendations are for fibrocystic breast disease that has been diagnosed by a qualified medical practitioner.

CANCER

DEFINITION

Cancer is an abnormality of body cells that have escaped from controlled behavior patterns. Atypical cellular growths spread to other areas and proliferate, ignoring the normal signal to stop growing and manifest themselves as malignant tumors. These tumors eventually impinge on glands and organs, causing their destruction. The degenerative process of cancer causes the deterioration of bones, lymph and blood.

CAUSES

The orthodoxy has not determined a cause for cancer and is just beginning to recognize that major carcinogens are environmental factors, diet and stress.

Holistic and natural healing physicians and scientists, through years of clinical and laboratory studies, have determined that toxins which have not been eliminated from the body destroy and weaken the DNA of the cell and immune system, allowing a virus to invade the inner workings of the cell and destroy it. In this process, the virus takes control of the cell by the manufacture of more viruses into it. When the cell no longer can contain the number of viruses, it explodes. Then these viruses migrate and attack other weakened cells. The cause of the weakened condition of the cell is determined by the lifestyle of the individual, including such factors as:

Smoking.

Alcohol consumption.

Toxic chemicals in the environment.

Pollutants.

Sunlight (ultra violet rays).

High tension wires.

Pesticides.

Standard American diet.

High sodium content of diet.

Insufficient amount of water consumed.

Insufficient sleep.

Lack of exercise.

Not eliminating toxins (bowel movements of insufficient amounts).

Imbalance of endocrine system.
Underactive thyroid.
Emotional stress.

Cancer patients share several common personality traits. They are often found to be:
Perfectionists.
Overachievers.
The type person who holds things in.
Self-debasing.
Putting everyone else first.
Putting self last.
Self-sacrificing.
The type person who wants to control.
The type person who needs cancer for attention.
Those with a death wish.

CONVENTIONAL TREATMENT

Surgery.
Radiation.
Chemotherapy.
Antihormonal drugs.

PROBLEMS ASSOCIATED WITH CONVENTIONAL TREATMENT

Modern medicine has not had a significant cut in the death rate from cancer since the 1950s. The National Institute of Cancer statistics show cancer is being treated better than it actually is. In the last 15 years, there has actually been a 5 percent increase in the death rate from cancer.

Surgery—Excising the so-called tumor, thinking the surgeon "has it all" is not a scientific determination. Cancer is not a localized affliction. It is a systemic disease which travels throughout the entire body. Removing a lump, organ or other bodily part and believing the cancer is no longer present is foolhardy because, in certain cases, the cancer will return in another area of the body (metastasis).

Surgical procedures in cancer patients are slow healing because of the weakened and depressed condition of the patient. Under conditions where the immune system is normal, healing will occur. However, if the immune system is depressed, which it usually is in cancer patients, healing will be compromised and further degeneration of overall health takes place.

Many drugs used in conjunction with the surgery further depress the immune system. In any surgical procedure, there is formation of scar tissue, and if it develops in a vital area or near organs or glands, it may eventually impinge on these organs, causing their dysfunction, since toxins accumulate in scar tissue and tightening occurs in those areas.

Radiation—X-rays have the potential to destroy DNA in the cell. An accumulation of years of different types of X-rays, such as dental, chest, those taken for fractures, mammograms, etc., culminate in a high degree of destruction. Radiation therapy is not selective enough and also affects areas adjacent to the ones being treated. For example, radiation for prostate cancer also damages the surrounding organs, including the large and small intestines, bladder and testes. Severe burns can also occur on the skin.

Chemotherapy not only destroys cancer cells. It also destroys other fast growing cells such as bone marrow, intestinal cells and hair. Side effects include peeling of skin, sores in the mouth, digestive problems such as vomiting, nausea, diarrhea, constipation and loss of appetite. The bone marrow which produces blood cells ceases to function properly in the manufacture of red and white blood cells. The immune system is so severely compromised that the patient is wide open to life-threatening infections. Hair loss is extremely stressful, especially to women. Many patients feel the side effects of this treatment are worse than the cancer, refuse to continue it and eventually expire.

Chemotherapy administered after radiation may be ineffective. Radiation causes fibrosis in tissues, thickening and hardening them. This makes the chemotherapy ineffective, but the orthodoxy continues to administer it.

Antihormonal drugs disrupt other hormones in the body which may lead to further imbalance and atrophy of the hormone producing glands.

ALTERNATIVE NATURAL REMEDIES

Prevention

Overweight people must adhere to a weight-lowering program since obesity causes over or underproduction of substances in the body that, in abnormal amounts, may cause malfunctioning of glands and organs.

Foods derived from animal sources have a tendency to weaken the immune system. Fat is difficult to digest and produces an overabundance and proliferation of highly poisonous toxins. Protein derived from animal sources breaks down into ammonia and nitrogen, toxic substances to the body.

Never eat foods cured with nitrites or charred or barbecued food. In the intestines, nitrates turn into nitrosamines, which are carcinogenic. Take vitamin C to avoid this phenomena. Charred or broiled foods drip their fat into the flame, pick up hydrocarbons and become benzine pyrine, a carcinogen, which enters the food that is being barbecued and subsequently consumed.

Drink only certified spring water or steam distilled water.

Tap water contains chlorine to destroy negative bacteria. However chlorine cannot differentiate between good and bad bacteria in the body and has the potential to destroy friendly bacteria.

Fluorine, which is a prescription drug that should be administered according to body weight, has been added to the water supply without our consent. A 175 pound adult and a 35 pound child who drink the same amount of tap water daily receive different proportions of fluorine in their bodies. The child gets a much higher percentage of fluorine per pound of body weight. This can have a deleterious effect in later life since fluorine, in addition to hardening teeth, also affects other tissues and may harden those that should remain soft.

Water pipes in the home are usually made of copper and have lead-soldered joints. Significant amounts of these metals leach into the water due to the acidic reaction of the chemicals added to the drinking supply. Too much lead in the body causes lead poisoning. In large amounts, copper may cause heart arrythmia and have a deleterious effect on red blood cells. Chlorine added to drinking water changes to tri halo methane, a carcinogenic chemical.

Avoid fish from polluted waters such as lakes, bays, rivers and seacoasts. Cold water, deep sea fish are the best. These include mackerel, halibut, sardines, salmon, tuna, flounder and orange roughy. Certified farmed fish are usually safe.

Diet

High rates of particular kinds of cancer can depend upon lifestyle and cooking methods. For instance, high rates of stomach cancer in Japan are attributed to the use of asbestos grills. The Japanese also filter sake through asbestos filters.

People living in countries with high dairy consumption have high rates of breast cancer. Populations, such as Seventh Day Adventists and strict vegetarians, whose diet is low in animal protein and high in complex carbohydrates, have the lowest incidences of cancer.

A strict macrobiotic regime, while helpful, is difficult for many people to follow. Try to eat as many macrobiotic foods as possible.

The largest portion of the diet should consist of organic vegetables, fruit, whole grains, starchy vegetables, nuts and seeds, tofu, tahini, hummous, miso soup, green tea, brown rice, and sea vegetables such as kelp, dulse, nori, etc.

Cruciferous vegetables such as broccoli, cauliflower, cabbage and Brussels sprouts produce an anti-cancer type substance.

Shitake and Reishi mushrooms stimulate the immune system and raise the T-cell count.

Eat at least ten almonds daily. They contain cyanide which is an anti-cancer ingredient.

Apricot pits (the interior of the seed, not the shell itself). This is where Laetrile (B17) is derived.

Pureed asparagus, four tablespoons daily. This is high in folic acid and sulphur which, when combined with vitamin A (Beta carotene), acts to deter the growth of some cancerous tumors.

Supplements

Cartilade, according to label. This substance is made from shark cartilage and severs the blood supply to the tumor, causing its death.

Squalene, for external use, aids in the healing process of skin damaged from the sun.

Vitamin A Beta carotene, 25,000 I.U. four times daily, stimulates the immune system and destroys free radicals.

Vitamin C, 50,000 to 100,000 mg. daily, administered intravenously by physician for a two week period (to bowel tolerance). When the patient develops diarrhea, the body no longer needs this amount of vitamin C and the amount should be decreased by 10 percent. Then switch to vitamin C (ascorbate) orally and take to bowel tolerance. Vitamin C helps prevent the oxidation process which can block cancer development. The last stage of cancer is scurvy, and Vitamin C can prevent scurvy.

Vitamin E, 800 IU. daily. Start with a a smaller dose and gradually work up to the 800 IU.

Selenium, 200 mcg. three times daily.

Glutathione, 500 mg. twice daily.

N-Acytal Cysteine, 500 mg. twice daily. This has a faster assimilation rate than L-Cysteine.

Oxynutrients by Allergy Research. This a highly effective antioxidant consisting of Germanium, CoEnzyme Q10, Dimethyl glycine (B15 or Pangamic acid), L-Carnitine, Ascorbyl Palmate Vitamin C (a fat soluble form of Vitamin C absorbed by body fat, an area not reached by water soluble Vitamin C), Gamma-oryzanol and Inosine. Take according to directions on label.

Hydrogen peroxide gel or liquid drops supply more oxygen to the system. The gel can be rubbed into the soles of the feet and the palms of the hands. The drops are a 35 percent solution that should be taken in water according to the directions on the label. According to the studies of Otto Warburg, who was awarded the Nobel Prize twice, cancer cells exist in an anaerobic environment. Their ability to live on oxygen has diminished, and they have derived a way to exist on the fermentation from anaerobic cells (basically sugar). Therefore, incorporating extra oxygen into the body may help in the destruction of the cancer virus.

Pancreatic enzymes taken between meals have the ability to break down the protein coating of the virus. With meals, they act as a digestive enzyme. Take according to directions of experienced holistic physician, and be sure they are from a reputable company as some sources have been contaminated.

Bromelain, 500 mg. three times daily, has the ability to destroy the virus after its protein coat has been absorbed by the pancreatic enzymes.

Vitamin B17 (Laetrile), dosage according to label, has the ability to destroy the virus after its shell has been absorbed, and it also helps control pain from cancer. It does not cure cancer, but can stop it from spreading.

Aloe vera gel, 2 ounces three times daily (keep refrigerated).

Green juices from alfalfa sprouts, wheat grass and blue green algae act as a blood cleanser and enhancer. Chlorophyll and human blood share some similar constituents. They have almost the same molecular configuration.

Extract of Venus Fly Trap and Live Cell Therapy are two methods being used by physicians in Germany.

Herbs

Chapparal is high in sulphur, has anti-tumor properties and is a painkiller.

Mandrake destroys cancer cells. Use with caution and do not use this herb if pregnant.

Periwinkle has shown promising results for chorio carcinoma and Hodgkin's Disease,

Pau D'Arco (Taheebo) has virus killing properties and is one of the strongest immune system stimulants.

Violet can be used internally and externally for tumors and malignant growths.

Echinacea, golden seal, dandelion root and ginseng all act as blood purifiers and detoxifying agents.

Saw palmetto berries can block the conversion of overproduced testosterone to its more potent form, Dihydrotestosterone, a carcinogen. It also prevents the hormone from binding to cellular receptors which could initiate prostate cancer.

Amino Acids

L-Methionine, 500 mg. twice daily on empty stomach, detoxifies environmental pollutants and radiation, reduces estrogen to less active estradiol and promotes antibody production.

L-Argenine, 1000 mg. three times daily on empty stomach, promotes wound healing and moderates the immune response through the thymus.

L-Glutathione, 500 mg. twice daily on empty stomach, stimulates the immune system, reduces production of free radicals and prevents overoxidation of cellular membranes.

L-Phenylalanine, 500 mg. four times daily on empty stomach, stimulates endorphins for reduction of pain.

Adjunctive Methods

Hyperthermia, the raising of body temperature to 107 to 108 degrees, selectively kills cancer cells while leaving normal tissue unharmed. This must be performed by a competent physician who is well experienced in this form of cancer therapy.

Breast surgery should not be scheduled from day 3 to 12 of the menstrual cycle since extra estrogen is produced at that time. Studies have shown that women whose surgery is performed day 13 to 32 of the menstrual cycle have higher survival rates.

Hydrazine sulfate. This is a prescription drug which prevents an enzyme from converting lactic acid to glucose. Normal cells exist aerobically (on oxygen). Abnormal or cancer cells exist through the process of fermentation which means they derive their oxygen from the breakdown oxygen of glucose. This fermentation does not allow the cell to derive the full amount of oxygen needed to exist in a healthy state.

DMSO (Dimethylsulfoxide). In leukemia the body is overwhelmed with immature white cells. In its attempt to compensate for this, the body produces even more of these immature white cells. DMSO aids in the maturation of these cells to their adult form.

CoEnzyme Q10, 30 mg. three times daily. The chemotherapy drug, adriamycin, depletes CoEnzyme Q10 from the body and may cause serious heart ailments. Replenishing CoEnzyme Q10 strengthens the heart.

Flutamide deactivates testosterone in cases of prostate cancer. Conventional medical treatment is castration and/or estrogen (female hormone) therapy, both of which deactivate testosterone, the male hormone which stimulates the growth of prostate cancer, but have disastrous side effects.

Clodronate for bone cancer (generally metastatic). This drug stops the outflow of calcium from bone, reduces pain and the spread of the cancer.

Alpha Interferon, 200 units orally, may be more effective than the orthodoxy's system of starting with a high dosage (3 million to 30 million units). High dosages have been proven to cause serious negative side effects.

Dr. Lawerence Burton's immuno augmentation therapy triggers action of antibodies that kill tumor cells.

Dr. Kelley's Treatment is a non-specific metabolic therapy consisting of:

1. Pancreatic enzymes which are able to destroy the shell of the virus.

2. Intense detoxification program of daily coffee enemas and liver and kidney flushes. (Coffee enemas should not be used if the patient has a colostomy).

3. High nutritional supplement approach.

4. Strict diet consisting mainly of fruits, vegetables, whole grains, complex carbohydrates, nuts and seeds and certain selected animal proteins.

5. Daily vegetable and juice regimen.

Liposoam therapy, used by Dr. Hans Neiper of Germany. Dr. Neiper mixes chemotherapy medication with lipospheres (little fat particles) so that only the tumor cells pick up the chemotherapy. This protects healthy tissue from exposure to the chemotherapy.

To learn more about these treatments and where they can be obtained, read the book, *The Third Opinion* by John Fink.

Meditation, imagery, affirmations, biofeedback and hypnotism are excellent adjuncts. Books, videos and classes are widely available.

Philosophical Statement

Cancer in the United States has been treated with respect to destroying the symptom and not addressing the underlying cause which is a depressed immune system. The toxins that accumulate in an unhealthy patient depress the immune system to such a degree as to render it extremely ineffective. These toxins which are the by-product of an unhealthy lifestyle are not in any way addressed by the orthodoxy. They believe that by excising the tumor and/or lymph nodes and giving radiation and chemotherapy that the disease is destroyed.

Cancer is not a localized disease. It is in every cell of the body and, therefore, each cell must be cleansed of the cancer virus or the disease will return in due time. Alternative therapy practitioners address this through detoxification programs. Chemotherapy destroys healthy cells as well as diseased cells. The diseased cells are destroyed but not eliminated fast enough, and when these remnants are left in the body, they cause a gangrenous condition to pervade from the dead matter. If the immune system exists in this state for an undue length of time, it is severely compromised to the degree of not having the ability to eliminate the disease, and other ailments are contracted. In holistic medicine, these toxins are eliminated by the detoxification program.

The emotional aspects of cancer are not addressed to their full potential by the orthodoxy. Cancer starts from a depressed immune system, which may have been caused by emotional stress. The everyday pressure of just existing in our society can be overwhelming. Our society pushes each individual to be number one. Not everybody has the potential or capability to arrive at the top. Striving to go beyond one's limitations leads to metabolic breakdown of the immune system and eventual self-destruction. Those who reach only what they consider to be secondary status in our society are considered failures because they did not achieve higher goals.

Typical cancer personalities feel like failures and try to overcompensate by doing more for others while wishing these others would do more for them. They constantly overextend their limitations by striving to be what they cannot. In their efforts to help others, their own survival is compromised.

CARPAL TUNNEL SYNDROME

DEFINITION

The wrist is a "U" shaped cradle of bones with the carpal ligament stretched across the open part of the "U" forming a tunnel. When this tunnel becomes smaller, the median nerve which runs through it, becomes compressed, causing pain, tingling and numbness in the hand.

CAUSES

Repeated wrist movements such as those performed by pianists, carpenters, typists, computer operators and people who knit and crochet can lead to:

Fluid in the canal, which increases in volume causing pressure on the nerve.

Rheumatoid arthritis, which causes the bones to thicken, leading to narrowing of the canal.

Tenosynovitis, a chronic inflammation of the membranes around the tendon.

CONVENTIONAL TREATMENT

Anti-inflammatory drugs.

Surgery.

Braces and splints.

PROBLEMS ASSOCIATED WITH CONVENTIONAL TREATMENTS

Cortisone weakens the adrenal glands by slowing down the body's production of its own hormone. Given over long periods of time, the patient can form an addiction as bodily functions become dependent on it. The adrenal glands have a better opportunity to rebound if cortisone is given every other day. Additional side effects are bloating, weight gain with a moon-face appearance, retinal problems and cataracts. Cortisone also stops the absorption of protein, curtails production of male and female hormones, can cause hair growth in undesirable places in women and breast enlargement in males. Since it is a steroid, it suppresses the immune system and makes the body more susceptible to infections. Prolonged use can also lead to psychotic behavior.

Non-steroid anti-inflammatories can cause dizziness, nausea, headache, constipation, diarrhea and vomiting.

Surgery is expensive and treats only the symptoms without addressing the true cause of the disability. Scar tissue formed from the surgery attracts bacteria and fungus to the area.

Braces and splints become cumbersome and tend to weaken other areas of your wrist and hand.

ALTERNATIVE NATURAL REMEDIES

If you have carpal tunnel syndrome, you may have a deficiency in Vitamin B6 and B2. This deficiency inflames and causes swelling in your tendons and tissues. Why? Because in carpal tunnel syndrome, fluid accumulates in your wrist. But vitamins B6 and B2 naturally reduce this fluid retention and swelling.

Diet

Eat foods that produce B vitamins such as whole grains, fruits, vegetables, complex carbohydrates, nuts and seeds.

Avoid saturated fats, simple sugars, junk food, fried foods, fast food, alcohol and spices such as mustard, ketchup, hot peppers,and relish.

Supplements

Vitamin B6, 200 mg. three times daily (use pyrodoxal #5, phosphate form of B6, which has a higher assimilation rate than plain pyrodoxine. Supplementing with plain B6 will not be as effective).

Vitamin B2, 100 mg. three times daily. Vitamin B12, 500 mg. sublingually twice daily. Always take B12 in the sublingual form since it cannot get into the system from the stomach if the intrinsic factor is not present. This is a factor that lessens with age.

When taking high amounts of singular B vitamins, one should add a 50 mg. B complex once daily for balance.

Bromelain, 500 mg., twice daily on an empty stomach. Bromelain acts as an anti-inflammatory when taken without food. If taken with meals, it acts as a digestive enzyme and will not be incorporated into the body as an anti-inflammatory.

Omega 3 fish oil, 1000 mg. four times daily. Best form is the mint flavored liquid, 2 tbsp. twice daily.

Cartilade, 12 pills daily, is an anti-inflammatory.

Vitamin C (ester C), 1000 mg. three times daily, acts as a general overall antioxidant.

Magnesium citrate, 500 mg. three times daily, acts as a muscle antispasmodic.

Herbs

Comfrey, coltsfoot and watercress all reduce fluid retention.

Yucca is a precursor to synthetic cortisone. It enables your adrenal glands to produce and release their own cortisone into your system.

Hydrangea acts like cortisone.

Amino Acids

L-Taurine, 500 mg. three times daily on empty stomach, acts as a diuretic.

L-Glutamine, 500 mg. four times daily on empty stomach, reduces potassium sodium electrolyte loss which, if not curtailed, could lead to even more fluid retention in your wrist.

DL-Phenylalanine, 500 mg. four times daily on empty stomach, elevates endorphins, the body's painkillers.

Cataracts

DEFINITION

A loss of the transparency of the lens of the eye, a condition which impairs or destroys vision. There are several different types of cataracts.

Traumatic cataracts from a perforating injury.

Irradiation cataracts from exposure to certain rays.

Complicated cataracts from ocular disease.

Congenital cataracts due to impaired formation during fetal life.

CAUSES

Cataracts are caused by aging, injury, heavy metal poisoning, X-rays, eye infections, exposure to ultraviolet light and use of certain drugs such as steroids. In diabetics, glucose diffuses into the lens forcing the lens metabolism to shift to the sorbitol pathway. This forms large amounts of sugar alcohol, increasing the influx of fluid into the lens which stretches the fibers, causing metabolic damage. This can also occur in non-diabetics.

Cataracts can also be caused by the swelling of the lens and its individual fibers which is the end result of deficiencies of certain enzymes. Deficiencies of potassium, and glutathione deactivate the molecular pumping system of the lens between the sodium and potassium concentrations. The sodium accumulates in much greater concentrations than normal, leading to the attraction of fluid from the aqueous humor of the eye into its lens.

CONVENTIONAL TREATMENT

Surgery.

PROBLEMS ASSOCIATED WITH CONVENTIONAL TREATMENT

Although cataract surgery has come a long way and is a much simpler procedure nowadays, it still has possible deleterious side effects. The assumption that cataract surgery is 99 percent foolproof must be taken lightly because cataracts are found mainly in the geriatric age group. An older person's body does not have the recuperative power to bounce back quickly from any surgical procedure. Most elderly people are highly deficient in the needed vitamins and minerals, amino acids, essential fatty acids, carbohydrates, fats and proteins needed to stimulate a healthy body.

Complications of surgery include: glaucoma, macular edema, hemorrhage, uveitis (eye inflammation), retinal detachment, surgical trauma, dislocation and/or clouding of the intraocular lens implant. There are also side effects from the drugs used in conjunction with surgery.

This information is not designed to instill fear, but is for the purpose of enhancing the knowledge of this procedure. Fear comes from lack of knowledge. Individuals who know what to expect are better prepared psychologically.

ALTERNATIVE NATURAL REMEDIES

Diet

Apples, blueberries and coconuts are fruits that strengthen weak eyes.

Beets, broccoli, cabbage, carrots, onions, turnips, collards, romaine lettuce and watercress are vegetables that strengthen weak eyes.

Fresh carrot juice is high in Vitamin A.

Supplements

Vitamin C (Ester C), 2000 mg. three times daily, is an antioxidant providing internal protection from the potentially damaging effects of light. It also protects the lens protein from oxidation.

Potassium citrate, 500 mg. twice daily, is needed for the activity of a particular enzyme (aldose reductase) which transports sodium out and potassium into the lens. Sufficient potassium is needed to balance this integral sodium/potassium pump.

SOD, Superoxide dismutase in the form of Cell Guard by Biotec. This helps alleviate the overproduction of the superoxide free radical in the lens. This free radical is known to be extremely destructive to the lens. The superoxide radical can self-dismutate into hydrogen peroxide and hydroxide radicals. Hydrogen peroxide made in the system can be deleterious if not scavenged by the antioxidant vitamins C, A, E and selenium.

However, if applied externally or taken internally, hydrogen peroxide has the ability to break down into nascent oxygen, which gives more oxygen to the respiratory action of cell metabolism, therefore lessening free radical production. It is not the same as what is made in the body as the by-product of cell metabolism.

Bioflavanoids—Quercetin, 500 mg. four times daily, helps increase capillary strength and regulate absorption of nutrients into the lens. It also helps inhibit the enzyme, aldose reductase. If aldose reductase is decreased, then sorbitol, which is sugar alcohol, will not form and will not induce accumulation of fluid in the lens.

Vitamin B2, 100 mg. twice daily.

Inositol, 500 mg. three times daily.

Vitamin B6, 100 mg. three times daily.

Selenium, 200 mcg. three times daily.

Vitamin E, build up to 800 I.U. daily. Take capsules containing E oil. They are more effective than the dry form.

Vitamin A (Fish liver oil), 25,000 I.U. once daily.

Vitamin B2 (Riboflavin), 100 mg. twice daily.

Beta carotene, 25,000 I.U. four times daily.

Herbs

Chapparal acts as an antioxidant, rebuilds tissue and is high in potassium.

Eyebright stimulates your liver to cleanse your blood which relieves the conditions that affect the clarity of your vision.

Bilberry is relaxing to the eyes.

Amino Acids

Glutathione, 500 mg. twice daily on empty stomach, preserves the physiochemical balance of the proteins within the lens, maintains the transport pumps (sodium and potassium) and molecular integrity of lens fiber membranes. It also maintains proper energy production.

Adjunctive Methods

Palming—Close eyes as tight as possible without straining. Place cupped palms over eyes so there is total darkness. Energy circulating through the body into the arms and hands revitalizes diseased cells in the eyes. Do this for five minutes daily.

Sunning—With closed eyes face the sun in early morning, before 9 am. Start with 15 seconds and add 15 seconds daily until reaching 5 minutes. Then go into a shaded area and rest with closed eyes for 2 minutes.

Spheno Palatine Block opens circulation in your eye by blocking the autonomic nervous system. (Must be done by a Holistic Medical Doctor.)

I highly recommend reading *The Eyes Have It* by Earlyne Chaney. It is an excellent self-health manual for better vision.

Cholesterol (high)

DEFINITION

If high levels of cholesterol are in the bloodstream, they can become trapped on the inside walls of the arteries, especially the coronary arteries (atherosclerosis). When these arteries are clogged with cholesterol deposits, also known as plaque, they become narrow and deprive the heart muscle of necessary nutrients and oxygen. The volume of blood to other vital areas is also reduced.

HDL levels are an important indicator for those at risk of heart disease. This is considered to be the good cholesterol that carries the bad cholesterol back to the liver so it can be eliminated from the body. The higher the HDL, the lower the risk factor for heart problems.

Below 25, dangerous.

26 to 35, high risk.

36 to 45, moderate risk.

46 to 59, average.

60 and above, below average.

CAUSES

Diet—Overconsumption of foods with a high saturated fat and high cholesterol content, such as fatty meats, heavy cream, butter and eggs.

Too much sugar.

Undue high stress—This causes overproduction of adrenalin which is manufactured in the adrenal glands. Cholesterol is necessary for this process. Adrenalin is needed to give extra energy to certain parts of the body because of the stress response. Most hormones, including adrenalin, are manufactured from cholesterol. Therefore, when more adrenalin is needed, more cholesterol is needed.

Genetic Predisposition.

Diuretics—can raise cholesterol. Along with increased urinary output, diuretics also cause essential minerals to be excreted. Mineral loss causes undue stress on the nervous system, leading to an increased need for adrenalin.

Injectable insulin—can raise cholesterol if blood sugar drops too low, causing the body to compensate by producing adrenalin to rebalance the system.

Estrogen and progesterone (female hormones) are derived from cholesterol. Levels will rise in women who have difficulty converting cholesterol to estrogen and progesterone

CONVENTIONAL TREATMENT

Cholesterol lowering drugs such as Questron, Cholefribate and Lovastatin.

Oat bran and rice bran.

Reduction of animal fat consumption such as meat, eggs, cheese, butter, cream, highly saturated oils and commercial baked goods.

PROBLEMS ASSOCIATED WITH CONVENTIONAL TREATMENT

Cholesterol reducing medications work by slowing down the absorption of cholesterol into the bloodstream. This is detrimental because, in addition to retarding the absorption of cholesterol, they also interfere with the absorption of essential fatty acids and the fat-soluble vitamins A, D, E and K. In addition, they block the total production of cholesterol, which is dangerous since most cells are composed of cholesterol.

Brans—In order to to be effective, a large amount of bran has to be eaten. This can result in weight gain, gas and boredom. The main reason bran lowers cholesterol is because people eat it instead of bacon and eggs.

ALTERNATIVE NATURAL REMEDIES

Diet

Avoid sugars and saturated fats. Sugar raises cholesterol by a chemical reaction in the body. It turns into triglycerides (blood fats) which eventually convert to cholesterol. Saturated fats reduce the liver's ability to rid the bloodstream of cholesterol Avoid the following foods:

Cookies	Cake
Ice cream	Soda
Candy	Pretzels
Crackers	White flour
White sugar	Honey

Molasses	Syrup
Pizza	Hoagies
Hot dogs	Hamburgers
Junk food	Processed food
Fast food	Fatty meats
Cream chees	Lard
Heavy oils	Processed oils
Dairy products	Fried or scrambled eggs

Supplements

Garlic, 500 mg. four times a day.

Lecithin, 6 capsules (19 grains) or 2 tbsps. granules daily.

Borage oil, 240 mg. twice daily, or Evening primrose oil, 6 capsules daily.

CoEnzyme Q10, 30 mg. three times a day.

Fish oil, 2000 mg. eicosapentenoic acid.

Multi-mineral containing zinc, magnesium and potassium.

Vitamin C, 1000 mg. four times daily.

Lipotropic factor (choline, inositol and methianine).

Niacin, start by taking 500 mg. for four days and add 500 mg. after each four day period until you build up a dose of 3000 mg. Take with 100 mg. B complex in order to avoid imbalance of B vitamins. When taking this dose of niacin, blood must be checked every two months because high niacin dosages can cause side effects such as gout, depression, irregular heart beat, glaucoma, cataracts, ulcers and changes in liver enzymes and proteins. If taking 3000 mg. daily, be aware of these risk factors. Do not take niacin if you are taking medication for high blood pressure.

Herbs

Devil's claw capsules or tea.

Fenugreek capsules or tea lowers cholesterol.

Butcher's broom capsules or tea aids circulation.

Amino Acids

L-Taurine, 500 mg. three times daily on empty stomach, moderates cholesterol production and fat metabolism.

L-Threonine, per label, is essential for fat metabolism in the liver.

L-Carnitine, 500 mg. twice daily, enhances the breakdown of fatty acids into energy in the cells of your heart.

L-Glycine, 500 mg. three times daily, is a precursor of bile, which is formed from cholesterol in the liver. When bile attaches to fiber, it is eliminated from the body, lowering cholesterol levels.

Stress Reduction

When the stress level is up, the body requires adrenalin for extra energy for the "fight or flight response". This raises the cholesterol level since the adrenal glands need cholesterol in order to manufacture adrenalin.

Exercise

Exercise can reduce cholesterol levels. In fact, farmers have a high intake of saturated fats and cholesterol laden foods, yet have a low incidence of heart problems because of the constant physical exertion of their everyday work.

WHY THE BODY NEEDS CHOLESTEROL

It acts as an antioxidant which helps rid the body of free radicals (poisonous by-products of cell respiration).

It is necessary for the production of bile.

It is needed as an ingredient in the membranes of all cells.

It is needed for production of brain neurons.

The body manufactures from 1200 to 2000 mg. of cholesterol daily for everyday activity, and it will make this amount of cholesterol no matter how much dietary cholesterol is consumed. In fact, for every 1 mg. of dietary cholesterol consumed, the liver produces 2.2 mg. less of manufactured cholesterol.

CHRONIC FATIGUE SYNDROME

DEFINITION

Devastating daily fatigue to the degree of incapacitation. The patient does not have enough energy to exist in a normal everyday fashion. For example just the act of brushing the teeth could use up the entire amount of reserve energy, exhausting the patients to such a degree that they must rest afterwards. Holding a job is next to impossible, and the condition can go on for years and eventually lead to such debilitation that depression and other side effects occur.

So far the orthodoxy has not found any treatment or method leading to remission. In fact they do not even recognize it as an established disease. Yet at this time, millions of people in the United States live with this disease and are so debilitated that they have lost all hope for recovery.

CAUSES

The function of the immune system is in such a depressed state that it can not supply the needed antibodies for normal protection of the body against the invasion of bacteria, viruses, pathogens and fungi. The immune system is further aggravated by the accumulation of toxins and other poisonous materials incorporated into the body from pollution and chemicals in food and water. Emotional states such as depression and anxiety, along with medication and lifestyle excesses add to the problem.

Many individuals are not aware of items in the house that have toxic effects. Rugs contain formaldehyde. Chemicals such as PBC and dioxin are in construction material. Chloro-fluoro-carbons are emitted from air conditioner and refrigerator units. These are the same chloro-fluoro-carbons that destroy the ozone cover of the earth. Detergents stored under the kitchen sink outgas. Chemicals are in cosmetics. Chlorine and fluorine are in the water supply. Outgassing occurs from automobiles if garage doors are closed too soon after parking. The gasses seep into the house. After putting cars in the garage the doors should remain open for at least 30 minutes.

The Epstein Barr virus, herpes virus, candida and food allergies and intolerances can cause chronic fatigue.

CONVENTIONAL TREATMENT

Stimulants such as caffeine.

PROBLEMS ASSOCIATED WITH CONVENTIONAL TREATMENT

Caffeine destroys pepsin in the stomach and interferes with normal digestion and absorption. Caffeine is an alkaloid, which is a vegetable poison.

ALTERNATIVE NATURAL REMEDIES

Low blood sugar (hypoglycemia) should be addressed since low blood sugar leads to fatigue. A six hour glucose tolerance test should be performed to determine blood sugar levels, insulin levels and whether patient is a potential diabetic.

Diet

It is very important to eat foods that do not cause fatigue. Eliminate anything difficult to digest such as refined foods, sugary foods, fried foods, preserved foods and smoked foods.

Avoid alcohol.

To strengthen the immune system, eat whole grains, brown rice, nuts, seeds, sea vegetables such as dulse, nori, kelp and arame.

Shitake and Reishi mushrooms stimulate the immune system and raise the T-cell count.

Eat complex carbohydrates in the form of fruits, green vegetables, whole grains, nuts, seeds and starchy vegetables that grow underground.

Drink distilled water.

Do not use microwave ovens. They destroy vitamins and enzymes. Food with bones does not cook evenly and pathogens can proliferate and cause disease.

Supplements

Vitamin C. In extreme cases, in order to get the high amount required, it is best given intravenously by a holistic physician. If this therapy is unavailable in your area, use vitamin C powder. Start with 5000 mg. daily and work up to bowel tolerance (when diarrhea occurs). Then cut down the amount (usually by 10 percent) until normal bowel function returns.

Vitamin A, Beta carotene, 25,000 I.U. four times daily.

Vitamin A, fish liver oil, 25,000 I.U. twice daily.

Vitamin E, start with 400 I.U. and gradually build up to 1200 I.U.

Selenium, 200 mcg. twice daily.

Iodine (kelp), 150 mg. three times daily, helps production of thyroxine in the thyroid.

Zinc picolinate, 50 mg. twice daily.

Multi-mineral, as directed on label.

B complex, 100 mg. twice daily.

The following are oxygenating supplements:

Germanium, 100 mg. twice daily. (Take more if affordable. This supplement is very expensive.)

CoEnzyme Q10, 30 mg. three times daily.

Dimethyl glycine, 125 mg. twice daily.

Octocosanol, a wheat germ derivative, 1 mg. three times daily.

The following are anti-inflammatory supplements:

Bromelain, 500 mg. twice daily between meals.

Garlic capsules, 500 mg. four times daily.

Gamma lineolenic acid (borage oil), 240 mg. three times daily.

Pantothene (B5), 300 mg. three times daily.

The following are liver cleansers:

Red clover combination.

Silymarin (milk thistle).

Herbs

Immuno aid combination by Nature's Way.

Pau D'Arco.

Echinacea.

Ginseng strengthens stress defense mechanisms.

Gotu Kola feeds brain and helps relieve mental fatigue.

Fo-Ti.

Guarana is a stimulant.

Super Pep (available in health food stores).

Amino Acids

L-Glutathione, 500 mg. twice daily on empty stomach, for free radical scavenging.

N-Aceytl Cysteine and L-Methionine, 2 capsules daily, clears out heavy metals and toxins from the bloodstream (acts as chelators).

L-Taurine, 500 mg. four times daily, moderates blood sugar levels.

Aspartic acid, per directions on label, aids in energy production.

L-Glutamine, 500 mg. four times daily on empty stomach, aids energy release in brain.

L-Alanine, per directions on label, is a major energy precurser.

L-Lysine, 500 mg. twice daily on empty stomach, reduces the inflammatory response of antibodies.

CONSTIPATION

DEFINITION

A sluggish condition of the bowels marked by irregular or difficulty in evacuation. The bowels should move at least once a day, and three movements, one after each meal, would be even better. Toxins that accumulate without being evacuated cause an imbalance in the bacterial flora of the colon and may stimulate disease.

CAUSES

The colon is the storage area for undigested refuse from food. Fluid is extracted from the refuse and channelled back into the system so the body will not dehydrate. If initially there is not enough fluid, the stools will be hard and what fluid is present will return to the body, making the stools even harder. Hardness of the stool slows the peristaltic action, causing it to be less effective and the waste material to move too slowly. Peristalsis is the muscular contraction and expansion of the colon wall that moves the waste through the colon to the sigmoid, rectum and out the anus.

Certain medications can cause constipation. Iron pills and calcium require a high acid environment to be properly assimilated. Extra vitamin C helps to assimilate these supplements. Constipation can also be a side effect of analgesics, antidepressants and many prescription drugs.

Not going to the toilet when the urge occurs, worrying, nervousness and grief will tighten the bowels.

CONVENTIONAL TREATMENT

Stool softeners.
Laxatives.
Bulking agents.
Fiber.
Mineral oil.
Enemas.

PROBLEMS ASSOCIATED WITH CONVENTIONAL TREATMENT

The orthodoxy may not associate normal bowel movements with good health. After a period of time, the patient may overly rely on medication which eventually weakens the natural ability to initiate peristalsis and exercise the sphincter muscle to allow normal bowel movements.

Mineral oil can remove vitamins and minerals from the system because it coats the intestinal walls and interferes with the absorption of these nutrients.

ALTERNATIVE NATURAL REMEDIES

Diet

Two types of fiber are soluble and insoluble. Soluble fiber is broken down and digested. It aids in the absorption of bile in the colon. Extracts of this bile can be carcinogenic if too high a concentration accumulates in the colon. Insoluble fiber is the indigestible part of food that moves through the system without being absorbed. It has a cleansing effect on the walls of the colon, but does not necessarily remove fat and bile.

Eat high fiber foods such as miller's bran, available in health food stores, whole grains including flax seed, oats, buckwheat, brown rice, kasha, blueberries, watermelon and other fruits with their skins.

Add complex carbohydrate-type vegetables, like potatoes and yams with their skins, beets, carrots, and corn, which has one of the highest fiber contents of all the vegetables. Beans have a high fiber content, but they may produce flatulence if they are not soaked and well cooked. Beano, a new product, aids in the digestion of beans.

Sauerkraut has a high fiber content and helps normalize the intestinal flora.

Snack on nuts, seeds, prunes, figs, dates and raisins.

Add lots of garlic to the diet. The allicin in garlic stimulates the walls of the intestines.

Drink at least eight to ten glasses of liquid daily as a natural stool softener.

Take psyllium seed husks twice daily, morning and evening. Mix one tablespoon in an eight ounce glass of water, stir vigorously and drink immediately before it gels and becomes difficult to swallow. Then fill the glass with plain water and drink it. Psyllium seed husks purchased in a health food store are free of the additives, coloring agents and sweeteners present in commercial brands. Note—If you don't drink enough liquid during the day while taking psyllium, it will have the opposite effect.

Avoid sugary foods, spices and fried foods.

Supplements

Vitamin C, to bowel tolerance (when diarrhea occurs, this means the body does not need any more).

Magnesium oxide, 2000 mg. daily in divided doses.

Enteric coated acidophilus, 1 hour before each meal.

Multidigestive enzymes, 1 after each meal.

Herbs

Buckthorn.

Cascara sagrada increases secretions of stomach, liver and pancreas, aiding in the breakdown of food. It also cleanses the colon and helps rebuild tissues.

Mandrake.

Senna increases intestinal peristaltic movements. It should be taken with ginger or fennel to prevent bowel cramps.

Amino Acids

L-Histadine, 500 mg. twice daily, promotes digestive secretions in the stomach needed to break down food particles into their tiniest parts, and enables digestion to take place in the proper part of the intestinal tract, causing less distress in the colon area.

Adjunctive Methods

Do exercises to strengthen the muscles that help in the evacuation and elimination process, such as sit ups, walking and diaphragmatic breathing.

Colonics. In extreme cases of constipation, a series of colonics is recommended to loosen the accumulated debris which has adhered to the lining of the colon. These are performed by a therapist with a water circulating machine that allows continuous water flow in and out of the colon for an extended time, usually 30 minutes. Once cleansed, the colon works more efficiently.

Cystitis

DEFINITION

Cystitis is a bacterial infection of the bladder characterized by an urgent desire to urinate. An overabundance of negative bacteria accumulates in the urine and causes dysfunction in the walls of the bladder. Symptoms include pain in the lower abdomen and back, frequent urgent and painful urination, blood or pus in the urine and fever.

Bladder infections are much more common in women than men due to their anatomy. In men, a bladder infection may be a sign of a more serious problem such as prostatitis.

CAUSES

Bacteria migrate up the urethra into the bladder. This can be due to several factors:

Wiping genitalia from back to front.

Vaginitis and yeast infections.

Sexual intercourse.

Use of diaphragm.

Food allergies.

Drugs and radiation.

Irritation from medical instruments used for diagnostic purposes.

Following catheterization.

CONVENTIONAL TREATMENT

Antibiotics.

PROBLEMS ASSOCIATED WITH CONVENTIONAL TREATMENT

Although antibiotics may relieve the condition, they do not address the cause, and cystitis has a propensity to recur. Antibiotics can cause yeast infections and inflame the problem.

ALTERNATIVE NATURAL REMEDIES

Diet

Asparagus stimulates kidney function.

Cherry juice helps relieve infections and stop frequent urination.

Cranberry juice. (Buy in health food store. Commercial brands contain too much sugar.) Cranberries contain quinic and benzoic acids as well as bacteriostatic substances that pass unchanged through the kidneys and urinary tract. Cranberry juice raises the acidity of the urine, creating an unfavorable environment for pathogenic bacteria.

Cucumbers, asparagus, parsley, watermelon and watercress stimulate kidney action and help flush out impurities and cleanse the system.

Avoid caffeine, alcohol, spices and carbonated beverages.

Drink steam distilled water, 8 to 10 glasses daily.

Supplements

Vitamin C, 1000 mg. four times daily, acts as a diuretic.

Vitamin B6, 100 mg. three times daily, acts as a diuretic.

Zinc picolinate, 50 mg. twice daily for infections.

Vitamin A Beta carotene, 25,000 I.U. twice daily.

Vitamin A, fish liver oil, 25,000 I.U. twice daily.

Acidophilus, enteric coated, 1 three times daily before meals.

Herbs

Corn silk clears the bladder of bacteria and reduces spasms.

Juniper berries aid in restoring kidney function.

Marshmallow root makes the urine more acidic and inhibits bacterial growth.

Dandelion tea helps relieve bladder discomfort.

Couch grass has a beneficial effect on the urinary system.

Uva ursi strengthens and tones urinary passages.

Amino Acid

GABA (Gamma aminobutyric acid), 500 mg. twice daily, moderates smooth muscle response in the genitourinary tract.

Adjunctive Methods

Urinate when you have the urge. Holding it in increases the risk of infection.

Wipe the genital area from front to back to avoid contamination.

Wear all cotton underclothes.

Women should drink water and empty their bladders before and after intercourse.

Women who use a diaphragm and suffer from repeated bladder infections should consult with a gynecologist about changing their method of birth control.

DEPRESSION

DEFINITION

A no-hope attitude and outlook and/or a feeling of despair. There are two types of depression: lethargic and high anxiety. Symptoms include fatigue, sleep disturbances, eating disorders, aches and pains and feelings that life has no purpose. Severely depressed people may consider suicide.

CAUSES

A negative interpretation of a situation or the environment.

A pessimistic outlook.

A deficiency or overproduction of neurotransmitters (mood altering chemicals).

Cerebral allergies. Certain foods or environmental pollutants can cause an allergic reaction in the brain.

Side effects of medication.

Pressures of life—marriage, workplace, lifestyle.

Alcoholism.

Drug addiction.

Demanding too much of self.

An unhealthy diet which can lead to deficiencies of amino acids, which are the precursors of neurotransmitters.

Low blood sugar.

CONVENTIONAL TREATMENT

Anti-depressant medicines.

Psychoanalysis.

Psychotherapy.

Behavioral therapy.

Electric shock therapy.

PROBLEMS ASSOCIATED WITH CONVENTIONAL TREATMENT

Medicines can block the under or overproduction of certain neurotransmitters, but any drug that is not natural eventually builds up since the body has no control over how much is taken in. When the body produces its own necessary medication, it only makes enough to satisfies its needs. This is known as the body's natural feedback system. Medication introduced into the body can build up too much, and undesirable side effects can occur such as:

A breakdown of one or more parts of any bodily function.

Cataracts.

Nausea.

Liver problems.

Headaches.

Diabetes.

If a poll were taken of the entire population who have undergone psychoanalysis, more than likely the majority would say they were not any better than before they started treatment. My own clinical experience over the past 15 years shows that depressed clients fall into the trap of relying too much on the therapist. In the long run this becomes a crutch and if the therapist is not available, the patient becomes even more depressed.

Most therapists do not have the innate ability and street sense to specifically ascertain the individual's main problem. They seem to use the same method of treatment on all patients. Each individual is unique and different and should be treated accordingly. Their method generally fails because the individuality of the person is not addressed.

In addition, the high cost of therapy is not affordable to lower income patients, whose depression is as real as that of the wealthy. Yet, depression in low income people is handled differently because of the cost factor. Many of these people are treated in clinics that do not have staff with the expertise to handle this type of problem.

Electric shock causes a change of the electrical energy in certain areas of the brain. In some instances this has to be made higher or lower due to either deficiency or overproduction of brain activity. The outcome is not always positive due to the complex activity of the brain which is unknown in depth to most of the medical profession.

ALTERNATIVE NATURAL REMEDIES

A holistic approach which entails not just psychotherapy, but the complete involvement of all aspects of the body, mind and spirit.

Body—A healthy outlook towards the foods, water and nutrients the body takes in.

Mind—A change in the philosophical outlook that people are conditioned to believe. Children are taught by two parents, who in most cases are complete opposites (which is what attracted them to each other in the first place). The children are caught in the middle and when drawn more to one parent, start to suffer guilt feelings about the other. It seems that people spend the rest of their lives, after age six, trying to get over the damage done during those years. This process is ongoing throughout life, unless changed through meditation, biofeedback, affirmations or imagery.

Spirit—Some individuals have the innate ability, through an unknown metaphysical phenomena deep in the spirit, that allows them to be able to visualize what they need to do to change their destructive patterns. These people have the luxury of knowing that, if they do not change, they will never be satisfied with themselves or anyone else. Through some unknown ability, they are convinced they must seize the moment and they are blessed with the insight to know when that moment arrives.

The insecurities people carry prevent them from having a back-up in cases of emergency. They are the type who step over the line in all relationships, jobs and objects. The insecurities force them to overcompensate in their relationships because they have a feeling of inadequacy. They overdo for others, which in turn activates a selfishness in these others.

Every pleasure in life has a price that must be paid, but when the time comes for this payment, a person may rebel. Many are under the delusion that life should be a happy state and never a sad one. People are taught that sadness, unhappiness, pain, etc. is not good. Therefore, they become depressed when misfortunes are encountered. Realistically, adversities are not negative. In fact, I perceive them as positive because they aid in strengthening us for future adversities.

The true statement should be that sickness and pain is a friend, not an enemy, but since everyone is taught the opposite, they continue along the premise of negativity. Actually adversities are warnings, without which people would never be able to prepare themselves for the oncoming battle. If changes in lifestyles and habits are not made, the negativity of the past will continue into the future.

Diet

The diet should consist mainly of protein and complex carbohydrates consisting of nuts, seeds and grains. It is important to eliminate sugar and any foods that convert to sugar such as fruit, juices, dried fruit, alcohol and starchy vegetables. Avoid all simple sugars plus anything ending in "ose" or "tol" such as mannitol, xylotol, dextrose and sucrose.

In abundance, sugar seems to give a quick energy burst, but the high is followed all too quickly by a drop in blood sugar levels (hypoglycemia). Low blood sugar causes depletion of glucose from the brain leading to a dysfunction of brain activity, and depression may occur. Hypoglycemia is the opposite of hyperinsulinism. Sugar levels rise and rapidly fall below the normal glucose level, causing low blood sugar which depletes the body and brain of the glucose needed to feed the brain.

Caffeine causes the overproduction of adrenalin which can lead to mood swings. Alcohol can cause depression.

Supplements

Vitamin C (ester C), 3000 mg. daily.

Vitamin B1 (thiamine), 100 mg. (is called the morale vitamin).

Vitamin B3 (niacin), 100 mg. twice daily (may cause flushing).

Vitamin B6, 100 mg. twice daily (take pyrodoxal #5 phosphate which is easier to metabolize).

Vitamin B12 sublingual, 500 mg. twice daily, aids in the conversion of amino acids to their respective actions in the body.

Take one multi-vitamin/mineral combination daily when taking extra B vitamins to balance the remaining B vitamins.

Zinc picolinate, 30 mg. twice daily.

Copper, 2 mg. daily.

Magnesium citrate, 400 mg. three times daily, has an excellent calming effect.

Herbs

Gotu kola eases mental fatigue.

Ginseng boosts body energy to overcome depression and stimulates and improves brain cells.

Valerian root is a nerve tonic for tension.

Catnip is soothing to the nerves.

Hops produces a calming effect on the nervous system.

Skullcap relieves stress and aids sleep.

Amino Acids

L-Tryptophan, a precursor of niacin and serotonin, a calming neurotransmitter. There have been problems with contamination of this product, and it may not be available.

Melatonin is taking the place of L-Tryptophan. It is produced by the pineal gland and is a calming neurotransmitter.

L-Tyrosine is a precursor of thyroid and adrenal hormones, epinephrine, norepinephrine and dopamine, all mood levelers.

L-Taurine moderates blood sugar levels, aids in the action of insulin, and helps to produce the neurotransmitters.

L-Glutamic Acid aids in regulating brain cell activity.

L-Glutamine reduces craving for alcohol.

Gamma Aminobutyric acid (GABA) has a neuroinhibitory action that helps calm and relax the body and reduce depression.

Avoid L-Argenine, which aids in the release of insulin.

Note: Neurotransmitter levels in the blood should be tested. Otherwise there is no correct way to ascertain whether there is an imbalance in he brain.

Diabetes

DEFINITION

A metabolic disorder characterized by the decreased ability or complete inability of the body to utilize carbohydrates due to lower production of insulin. The major symptoms are excessive thirst, frequent urination, and increased appetite with weight loss. Other symptoms include muscle cramps, poor healing of wounds, impaired vision and itching.

In addition to blood sugar levels, diagnostic tests for insulin levels should be performed. These are:

C Peptide—Fasting.

C Peptide—24 hour urine.

Glucogan stimulated C Peptide.

CAUSES

Type 1 or juvenile diabetes is caused by the cessation of insulin production.

Type 2 or adult onset diabetes is caused by an insensitivity to the amount of insulin produced.

As a person ages, insulin production diminishes. If the sugar intake is the same or increases, the blood sugar will rise, and if the level gets too high, that in essence is diabetes.

Diabetes can lead to the gradual deterioration of eyesight and vision problems (diabetic retinopathy). It can cause circulatory problems in the lower legs which eventually become ulcerated and may lead to gangrene, necessitating amputation. Heart problems can occur due to the overproduction of insulin in those with adult onset diabetes. Insulin enhances growth of endothelial cells in the arteries, causing them to break down, leak and erode. This leads to atherosclerosis and blockage in the coronary and carotid arteries. Plaque forms to seal the eroded areas and eventually forms clots.

Patients with heart conditions who take calcium blockers should be aware that they also block calcium from the islet cells in the pancreas. Calcium is needed to release insulin from these cells.

Potassium depletion from diuretics impairs insulin release.

CONVENTIONAL TREATMENT

Juvenile diabetes—Insulin.

Adult onset diabetes—Oral blood sugar lowering pills (Diabenese), weight control and the ADA diet based on high complex carbohydrates.

PROBLEMS WITH CONVENTIONAL TREATMENT

Those with juvenile or Type 1 diabetes must take insulin in order to survive. Most diabetics take one long-acting dose and sometimes two shorter acting dosages during the day. A normal body produces high amounts of insulin before and during meals and production is usually low between meals and while sleeping. The best way to administer insulin so the body will feel like it is in a natural state is to take it 30 minutes before each meal along with small amounts between meals. Although this method may seem cumbersome, it is more efficient and effective in controlling and lessening the intake of insulin which is known to be a powerful destructive hormone to some body parts when it is overproduced.

Oral blood sugar lowering pills have a high failure rate, may cause premature death from cardiovascular disease and may have toxic effects on older people.

The high complex carbohydrate diet is not necessarily the best one for diabetics. All carbohydrates, whether simple or complex, convert into sugar (glucose), and since insulin is needed to convert glucose into energy, it is more sensible to decrease rather than increase the amount of carbohydrates ingested. Carbohydrates are not essential to the body. Essential nutrients are proteins and fats which convert to energy by metabolic means other than insulin action.

Some fats are essential, but I am not recommending a high fat diet. Enough fat is present in food after removing visible portions. Protein in the diet comes from fish, fowl, meat, dairy and eggs. Nothing is wrong with this type of food if it is obtained through organic sources. It is not the food that causes disease. The problem comes from chemicals added to the feed given to animals.

Certain ethnic groups such as Eskimos and Laplanders consume a diet consisting mainly of fat and protein from fish, seal, walrus and polar bear. Carbohydrates cannot grow in the North Pole. Until they enter civilization, Eskimos are one of the healthiest groups on the planet. Their average cholesterol is 135, they have no heart disease and the word "headache" is not even in their language.

Carbohydrates are strictly an energy producing food. The traditional theory is that if none are ingested, the individual would be deprived of an energy-producing food. This is not so. The body can produce energy from stored fat and protein, a process called gluconeogenesis. In addition, ketone bodies are broken down from the fat and converted into energy.

ALTERNATIVE NATURAL REMEDIES

Diet

Eat foods high in protein (one gram for every two pounds of body weight), low in carbohydrates and high in fiber. High fiber foods form a gel in the intestinal tract to trap sugar for a period of time so it will be more slowly absorbed into the intestines.

An alkaline rather than acid-producing diet is better for diabetics in extreme acidosis because it is a disease of overacidity. High acidity in the pancreas causes the destruction of insulin-producing beta cells, and when the system is overacidic, fats and proteins are not broken down properly. Acid-forming foods are grains, except for millet and buckwheat, all flesh foods and dairy products, eggs, nuts, except for almonds and Brazil nuts, and lentils. Alkaline type foods are all vegetables and fruits, millet, buckwheat, Brazil nuts and coconut. This low acid, high alkaline type diet only applies to diabetics in extreme acidosis. Those with moderate cases should follow the high protein, low carbohydrate diet.

Foods aiding in insulin production are as follows.

Raw foods stimulate the pancreas. 80 percent of the diet should consist of raw foods.

Cucumbers contain a hormone needed by cells of the pancreas to produce insulin.

Onions and garlic contain natural beneficial hormones.

Jerusalem artichokes stimulate insulin production.

String bean juice or string bean pod tea helps keep glucose under control.

A simple sugar not broken down by insulin is fructose (sugar from fruits) and, in moderate amounts, it can be utilized by diabetics.

Supplements

Chromium picolinate, 200 mcg. three times daily, is needed to activate receptor sites on cells. In most diabetics these cells do not open properly, thereby slowing down the amount of glucose and insulin entering them.

Zinc picolinate, manganese and magnesium citrate are essential in the breakdown of glucose into cell energy.

Zinc picolinate, 30 mg. twice daily.

Manganese, 25 mg. twice daily.

Magnesium citrate, 500 mg. twice daily.

Biotin, 1 mg. three times daily.

Inositol, 650 mg., two capsules three times daily. Seven percent of ingested inositol converts to glucose and helps take the load off the body's production of glucose. Coffee depletes the body's storage of inositol.

Potassium citrate, 500 mg., stimulates insulin production.

Vitamin C, 1000 mg. three times daily, stimulates insulin production.

Vitamin B1, 100 mg. twice daily.

Vitamin B2, 100 mg. twice daily.

Vitamin B5, 100 mg. twice daily.

Vitamin B12, 500 mcg. sublingual twice daily.

Cartilade, 12 a day for 3 weeks. Then cut back gradually until reaching a maintenance dose of 4 a day. This reduces bleeding of the cells in the retina (diabetic retinopathy) and prevents angiogenesis (production of unwanted blood vessels).

Herbs

Alfalfa.

Cayenne red pepper.

Dandelion root helps liver excrete stored glucose as glycogen.

Uva ursi is a remedy for excessive sugar.

Sinita organa (cactus plant) contains natural insulin.

Blueberry leaf.

Amino Acids

L-Glutathione, 300 mg. twice daily on empty stomach, aids as a glucose tolerance factor.

L-Glutamic acid, 500 mg. three times daily on empty stomach, aids in sugar and fat metabolism.

L-Glutamine, 500 mg. four times daily, reduces craving for sugar.

L-Lysine, 500 mg. twice daily, promotes insulin production.

L-Taurine, 500 mg. twice daily, potentiates the action of insulin in carbohydrate metabolism and moderates blood sugar levels.

L-Tryptophan, from foods such as turkey, pumpkin seeds, milk and cheese reduces carbohydrate cravings.

Exercise

Moderate exercise, such as walking or light calisthenics, increases the uptake of glucose by muscle cells which reduces blood glucose. Exercise also increases muscle mass, and a large muscle mass creates a greater need for energy even when not exercising. When the amount of glucose in the body is low, glycogen is activated from the liver to the bloodstream to be used as energy. Utilizing the energy tends to bring down high glucose levels.

Adjunctive Remedy

Zostrex cream (capsicum-cayenne red pepper extract), applied topically to areas of diabetic neuropathy, prevents your skin from atrophying and ulcerating.

Avoid

Stress, which causes the release of certain hormones, glucogan, cortisol and catecholamines. These inhibit insulin secretion and increase the production of glucose by the liver from glycogen reserves.

Cortisone, which is antagonistic to insulin.

Birth control pills, which affect carbohydrate metabolism in a negative manner.

Diuretics, which stimulate excretion of water and cause an increase in the concentration of glucose.

Digestive Disturbances

DEFINITION

The inability to break down food in the stomach and intestines, leading to disease, malnutrition and unmetabolized food.

CAUSES

Mastication, which is the breakdown of food by chewing, is not properly performed. Saliva contains an enzyme (amylase) which starts the digestive process. Food should be well broken down by the teeth and moistened with saliva before it is swallowed. A deficiency in salivary gland output may lead to a disruption of the initial breakdown process.

The esophagus, the tube from the mouth to the stomach, may not function properly.

As people age, there is a slowdown in production and potency of the digestive enzymes and hydrochloric acid in the stomach. Individuals who secrete low amounts of stomach acid are highly susceptible to polyps in the digestive tract. Indications of low stomach acid production are enlarged joints in the fingers, periodontal disease, plaque on the back of the teeth and bad breath in the morning.

There may also be a slowdown in the digestive enzymes produced in the pancreas, which are needed to break down fats, proteins and carbohydrates.

The liver's production of bile, which breaks down fats, is lessened.

The muscular action of the stomach and intestines (peristalsis) that pushes food along is weakened, due to a general overall depletion in body nutrients needed by the muscles.

Stress causes the overproduction of hormones which deactivate certain areas of the body to prepare it for the fight or flight response. The stomach and intestines are one of these deactivated areas. If digestion is in progress at this time, it will be interrupted by this phenomenon, leading to indigestion, heartburn, flatulence, belching and hiccupping.

Spicy type foods such as mustard, relish, ketchup and hot spices require higher amounts of enzymes to be broken down.

The natural enzymes present in food are destroyed if it is overcooked. This puts more of a burden on the body to produce enzymes.

Processed foods which contain chemical additives and preservatives are also difficult to break down.

Fatty foods use a higher amount of hydrochloric acid from the stomach, and this may cause heartburn.

Sugary type foods which take a high amount of insulin for breakdown disrupt the normal digestive process.

Swallowing air due to talking while eating can cause gas.

Drinking liquids during meals dilutes digestive juices.

Overly cold food causes contraction of the stomach lining, lessening the amount of digestive juices produced.

Overly hot food causes the stomach lining to expand and produce too many digestive juices.

Gallstones, which block the ejection of bile into the intestines, can slow down the breakdown of fats.

Overeating, eating too fast and poor food combining puts too much stress on the digestive process.

CONVENTIONAL TREATMENT

Antacids.

Antispasmodics.

PROBLEMS ASSOCIATED WITH CONVENTIONAL TREATMENT

Antacids drain hydrochloric acid from your stomach—thus preventing it from breaking food down to its necessary nutrients. The underproduction of the acids and enzymes leads to fermentation of the partially digested foods, producing gas. Antacids also contain aluminum, which may cause brain cell deterioration.

Antispasmodics can have serious side effects, both mental and physical. Older individuals should be especially careful when taking these drugs as they can worsen glaucoma, cause blurring of vision and difficulty urinating, especially in men with enlarged prostates.

ALTERNATIVE NATURAL REMEDIES

Eat slowly and chew food well.

Avoid discussing stressful topics while eating.

Avoid spicy foods.

Avoid processed foods.

Avoid fatty foods.

Avoid sugary food.

Avoid swallowing air. Do not talk too much while eating, and do not drink carbonated beverages.

Do not drink liquids 30 minutes before, 45 minutes after, or during meals. Never drink tea when consuming protein as it contains tannic acid which reduces the absorption of protein through the intestinal wall.

Avoid overly hot or cold foods.

Do diaphragmatic and abdominal exercises to strengthen the stomach muscles.

Be careful not to eat foods at the same meal that do not combine well with each other. Do not eat protein and starchy foods at the same time. Starches with greens or proteins with greens are acceptable combinations. Eat fruit separately, not with protein or carbohydrates.

Supplements

Digestive multiple enzymes, 1 or 2 with each meal.

Aloe vera gel, 2 tbsp. three times daily (store in refrigerator).

Acidophilus, enteric coated, 1 three times daily between meals.

Peppermint oil, according to directions on label.

Vitamin B complex, 50 mg. twice daily, aids digestion and helps break down carbohydrates.

Swedish bitters, per label, help produce hydrochloric acid in the stomach.

Herbs

Wormwood helps maintain proper stomach acidity.

Chickory.

Hops increases appetite.

Lemon grass.

Papaya has natural digestive enzymes.

Peppermint, a good stomach sedative.

Safflower strengthens your liver and helps alleviate gall bladder problems.

Saw palmetto enhances appetite.

Thyme, a general tonic with healing powers.

Ginger alleviates nausea.

Yarrow alleviates nausea.

Amino Acids

L-Histidine, 500 mg. twice daily on empty stomach, promotes stomach digestive secretions.

L-Glutamine, 500 mg. four times daily on empty stomach, has a calming effect on the stomach.

L-Taurine, 500 mg. three times daily on empty stomach, is a precursor of bile, improves digestion and ileal disorders and potentiates the action of insulin in fat metabolism.

L-Threonine, 500 mg. twice daily, is essential for fat metabolism in the liver.

L-Carnitine, 500 mg. twice daily on empty stomach, stimulates pancreatic and gastric secretions.

Dry Eyes and Dry Mouth

DEFINITION

Sjogren's syndrome is a condition where the fluids that lubricate the eyes and mouth cease to operate properly, thereby producing dryness and inflammation. It is related to rheumatoid arthritis, and may lead to secondary glaucoma, cataracts or degeneration of the eye because of inflammation. Dry mouth could be a factor in digestive disturbances since the enzymes in saliva aid in the breakdown of food.

CAUSES

Food allergies.

Side effects of medications.

Stress.

Female hormonal changes (menopausal).

Overproduction of (PGE 2) inflammatory prostaglandins. These are produced by toxins in the body which are derived from hydrogenated oils (particularly margarine) and the overconsumption of sugar.

Systemic yeast infection—Toxins escape from the colon and intestine into the bloodstream and may attack other parts of the body.

Parasites rob the body of nutrients and also can travel in the bloodstream throughout the body causing destruction of tissues.

Stones in the salivary glands can cause dry mouth.

Carotid artery occlusion (rare).

CONVENTIONAL TREATMENT

Anti-inflammatory drugs.

Eye drops.

Artificial tears.

Electrical stimulation.

PROBLEMS ASSOCIATED WITH CONVENTIONAL TREATMENT

Drugs address only the symptoms, not the cause of the condition. Anti-inflammatory drugs may cause liver problems, weight problems, bloating and cataracts.

Eye drops may cause stinging, burning, pain, blurred vision, increased sensitivity to light, itching, swelling, redness or overproduction of tears.

ALTERNATIVE NATURAL REMEDIES

Food and environmental allergy testing such as:

Cytotoxic—a microscopic examination of blood cells to determine the action of antibodies when food extract is added.

RAST (a blood test for food allergies).

Muscle testing by kinesiology (can be performed by holistic chiropractor).

Reducing stress levels allows less pressure on the glands that secrete the lubricating fluids for the eyes and mouth.

A healthy lifestyle including elimination of hydrogenated oils and sugars. Natural foods aid in the production of anti-inflammatory prostaglandins (PGE 1), which have a balancing effect on the system. Denatured foods cause the overproduction of inflammatory prostaglandins (PGE 2).

Diet

Dry eyes, if caused by a deficiency in oils, can often be relieved by consuming two tablespoons of flaxseed oil daily. This can be used in salad dressing. Other beneficial oils are canola, safflower and olive. (Keep oils refrigerated).

Avoid all foods that contain hydrogenated oils such as commercial baked goods, potato chips, commercial pop corn and margarine.

Eliminate saturated fats as they can cause the clogging of capillaries that feed the glands that produce lubricating fluids.

Avoid foods where hydrogenation is used as a preservative. Hydrogenation works by decreasing the oxygen content and can also steal oxygen from the bloodstream. Cells which depend on oxygen starve, do not operate properly and become dysfunctional.

Avoid sugars and sugar producing foods. These depress the immune system, affecting protective antibodies that ward off viruses and bacteria which can attack the lacrimal glands of the eyes and parotid or salivary glands of the mouth.

Drink fresh carrot juice which is high in Vitamin A.

Raw potato juice improves eyesight.

Sunflower seeds, apples, blueberries and coconut are all good for weak eyes.

Supplements

High vitamin/mineral combination, 1 daily.

Vitamin A, 25,000 I.U. fish liver oil, one daily.

Vitamin A, Beta carotene, 25,000 I.U. twice daily, aids in vision and healthy eyes.

Vitamin B6, 100 mg. twice daily, helps prevent infection of eyes.

Vitamin C, 1000 mg. four times daily, is a detoxifying agent and heals infections.

Vitamin D, 400 I.U. twice daily, works with Vitamin A for healthy eyes.

Vitamin E, 400 I.U., works in synergy with Vitamin A (helps activate each other).

Anti-inflammatory types are:

Pantothene, 300 mg. three times daily.

Fish oil, 1000 mg. capsules, six times daily.

Bromelain, 500 mg. twice daily.

Garlic, 500 mg. four times daily.

Vitamin B1, 200 mg. twice daily.

Gamma Linolenic acid, GLA in the form of Evening primrose oil, or borage oil which is more effective and less expensive. According to label.

Cod liver oil, 1 tbsp morning and evening on empty stomach. Keep refrigerated.

Magnesium citrate, 400 mg. three times daily, is an antispasmodic type supplement that prevents capillaries from going into spasm.

Herbs

Golden seal, a natural antibiotic for eye infections.

Eyebright, for healing and strengthening.

Bilberry, to strengthen your eyes.

Cayenne acts as a vasodilator for the microcapillary system and aids circulation.

Ginger removes congestion and relieves pain.

Passion flower helps inflamed eyes and relieves dim vision.

Amino Acids

L-Taurine protects eyes from toxins.

L-Histadine is a vasodilator.

L-Lysine reduces inflammation response of antibodies.

Adjunctive Remedies

Some natural tears (available over the counter for lubricating the eyes) that are preservative free and do not sting the eyes are:

Hypo tears.

Tears Natural.

Liquid tears.

Refresh tears.

For dry mouth, use of the Salitron, a device which delivers mild electrical stimulation to specific areas of the tongue, causing an increase in the flow of saliva. To order or receive information call 1-800-82-OASIS.

EMPHYSEMA

DEFINITION

Chronic obstructive lung disease. Abnormal swelling and destruction of the lung and sacks of the lungs leads to a loss of their elasticity, causing a decreased ability to utilize oxygen.

CAUSES

Smoking.
Air pollution.
Dust.
Bronchitis.
Asthma.
Other respiratory diseases.
Asbestos (work related).

CONVENTIONAL THERAPY

Anti-inflammatory drugs.
Antibiotics.
Portable respirators.
Inhalers (bronchodilators).

PROBLEMS ASSOCIATED WITH CONVENTIONAL THERAPY

All drugs address only the symptoms, not the cause of the condition. Anti-inflammatory drugs may cause liver problems, weight problems, bloating and cataracts. Antibiotics may have allergic type side effects, such as yeast infections, hives, itching, a rash and wheezing.

Respirators are very cumbersome. In severe cases of emphysema, a portable respirator may not be sufficient to aid breathing.

Use of inhalers can cause the natural breathing mechanism to atrophy to such a degree that the ability to breathe may become solely dependent on them. Inhalers have also been known to lead to stunted growth in children, peptic ulcers, convulsions, glaucoma, abnormal heart rhythm and possible death.

ALTERNATIVE NATURAL REMEDIES

Diet

Cayenne pepper, hot peppers, coffee, horseradish and mustard all act as vasodilators. (A word of caution—all may raise blood pressure).

Honey clears mucous and phlegm from the lungs and soothes coughing spasms.

Grape juice clears mucous and phlegm from the lungs.

Sour fruits such as pineapple and berries help dissolve mucous.

Barley water contains hordenine, which relieves bronchial spasms.

Raw onion acts as an expectorant. It is so potent that bronchial spasms can often be relieved by sucking on a slice of onion.

Supplements

Anti-inflammatory types are:

Pantothene, 300 mg. three times daily.

Fish oil, 1000 mg. capsules, six times daily.

Bromelain, 500 mg. twice daily.

Garlic, 500 mg. four times daily.

Vitamin B1, 200 mg. twice daily.

Gamma Linolenic acid, (GLA Evening primrose oil) according to label, or borage oil which is more effective and less expensive.

Cod liver oil, 1 tbsp morning and evening. Keep refrigerated.

Supplements for oxygenation are:

Germanium, 50 mg. three times daily minimum. This supplement is very expensive. If affordable, increase dosage to 500 mg. daily.

DMG, Dimethyl glycine, also known as B15 or Pangamic acid, 125 mg. twice daily.

CoEnzyme Q10, 30 mg. three times daily.

Vitamin E, 400 I.U. twice daily. This acts as a blood thinner, helps guard against air pollution and helps your body and lungs use oxygen more efficiently. Start out with a lower dosage and work up gradually to avoid raising blood pressure.

Vitamin A, Beta carotene, 25,000 I.U. 4 times daily.

Vitamin C, 1000 mg. to bowel tolerance (when diarrhea occurs), then cut back (until diarrhea stops) and maintain that dosage.

Multi-mineral, 2 daily.

Magnesium citrate, 400 mg. three times daily, acts as an antispasmodic and vasodilator.

Folic acid, 800 mcg, five times daily, helps strengthen lungs.

Herbs

Comfrey is protective to the respiratory system.

Ephedra is a decongestant.

Fenugreek expels phlegm and mucous.

Mullein has antibiotic properties for the respiratory system.

Slippery elm bark decreases inflammation.

Lobelia, a very important herb to relax and clear the air passages of the lungs.

Garlic acts as an antibiotic and helps dissolve mucous from the bronchial tubes.

Amino Acids

N-Aceytyl Cysteine liquifies mucous and loosens mucous plugs from the lungs.

L-Histadine acts as a vasodilator and reduces the tendency for allergy.

Adjunctive Methods

Stop smoking.

Do deep breathing exercises and upper body calisthenics.

Maintain normal weight.

Raise head of bed to help drain mucous while sleeping.

Use humidifier if environment is dry.

Keep windows open as much as possible in order to counteract indoor pollution.

Anise seed oil, 5 to 10 drops on 1 tsp of brown sugar three times daily, before meals, removes mucous.

ENDOMETRIOSIS

DEFINITION

A disease in which tissue from the lining of the uterus (the endometrium) implants elsewhere in the pelvic structures, usually on the ovaries, fallopian tubes, bladder or bowel wall. It causes lower back pain, excessive bleeding accompanied by the passage of clots, nausea, constipation and painful intercourse.

CAUSES

Proliferation of active estrogen which causes enlargement and expansion of the endometrium.

Birth control methods such as intrauterine devices, antispermacides and birth control pills. (In certain cases, birth control pills are prescribed for this condition because the estrogen in the pill tends to slow down the patient's active estrogen).

CONVENTIONAL TREATMENT

Antihormonal drug therapy.

Surgery (hysterectomy) or laser treatments to eliminate overgrowth of endometrium.

PROBLEMS ASSOCIATED WITH CONVENTIONAL TREATMENT

The treatments address symptoms rather than causes. After a hysterectomy you can suffer from dropped bladder, vaginal dryness, and nerve damage which can lead to urinary incontinence and bowel problems. Severing of muscles, ligaments and tendons may cause back problems. Your risk of a heart attack increases by three times. In addition, after a hysterectomy, women's bodies often enlarge to where they have to wear two sizes larger than prior to the surgery.

Antihormonal drugs cause an imbalance of other hormones. The body's feedback system ceases to function properly when synthetic hormones are taken. This can activate the overproliferation of unnatural estrogens which may lead to cancer. Hormones can also cause masculine characteristics such as deepening of the voice and excess facial hair growth.

ALTERNATIVE NATURAL REMEDIES

Since estrogen is a fat soluble hormone, it is stored in fatty tissue, so, with less body fat, smaller amounts will be present. If overweight, a weight loss diet is essential. The most effective way to lose weight is to adhere to a high protein, low fat, low carbohydrate diet. To aid weight loss, the following appetite suppressant supplements may be used:

L-Phenylalanine, 500 mg. four times daily on an empty stomach.

Guar gum powder in water, one half hour before meals.

Thermogenic tea one half hour before meals.

Diet

Avoid or cut back estrogen producing foods such as carrots, yams, pomegranate seed, legumes, endive, oatmeal, wheat germ, alfalfa, brewer's yeast, sunflower seeds and liver.

PABA or folic acid also produce estrogen. Avoid organ meats, asparagus, leafy greens, peanuts, mushrooms and whole grains. Do not use sunscreens containing PABA as it can be absorbed through the skin. If you use a multi-vitamin, be sure it does not contain PABA or folic acid.

Use dairy products, eggs and meats obtained from organic sources only, since most animals are raised on growth hormones which can affect the system. Make sure dairy products are non-fat since hormones store in fatty tissues, and abstain from cow's milk because it is loaded with hormones.

Supplements

Oxynutrients is a high antioxidant supplement containing coenzyme Q10, germanium, DMG, inosine, gamma oryzanol, L-Carnitine and ascorbal palmitate which is a fat soluble form of vitamin C that activates its antioxidant property in fatty tissue. Take as directed on label.

Lipotropic factor, 2000 mg. daily (product may come in different strengths: usually 3 capsules = 1000 mg. and 6 capsules would = 2000 mg.). Take twice daily with meals.

This is composed of choline, inositol and methionine and helps enhance the action of the liver to break down the active forms of estrogen (estradiol and estrone) into inactive estrogen (estriol). Therefore the cells are not overly activated to boost endometrial growth.

Herbs

Red clover combination enhances liver function.

Sarsaparilla helps regulate hormones.

Blessed thistle aids in menstrual disorders.

False unicorn helps uterine disorders.

Siberian ginseng corrects hormonal imbalances.

Red raspberry contains nutrients to strengthen the uterine wall. It decreases uterine swelling and prevents uterine hemorrhage.

Amino Acid

L-Carnitine, 250 mg. twice daily, enhances fat burning.

Adjunctive Modalities

Abstain from sexual intercourse during menstruation since coitus can push secretions back through the fallopian tubes into the pelvic cavity. Orthodox Jewish women and members of other societies with menstrual taboos have a low incidence of endometriosis due to sexual abstinence at this time.

An imbalance between estrogen and progesterone can cause the proliferation of endometrial growth. An excellent product for hormonal balance is Progestade. It is applied to the skin and eventually absorbed into the bloodstream. It is not available in stores but can be ordered by calling 1-800-648-8211 or by writing to Box 3427, Eugene, Oregon 97403.

EPILEPSY

DEFINITION

A disease characterized by seizures.

Two types of seizures are:

Simple partial, *i.e.* sensory, where a change in sensation occurs. There may be a loss of consciousness.

Convulsive seizures which are characterized by abnormal muscular behavior, unconsciousness, convulsions and sometimes loss of bladder control.

CAUSES

Seizures are caused by an electrical disturbance in the nerve cells in one section of the brain, resulting from factors such as hypoglycemia, tetanus, malnutrition, rabies, lead poisoning, meningitis, head injury, fever or infection.

Precipitating factors are tension, excitement, menstruation, fatigue, overconsumption of alcohol, overeating and environmental stresses. Artificial sweeteners may be associated with seizures.

Alcoholism in mothers while pregnant stops neurons (brain cells) from travelling to their designated areas in the fetal brain.

CONVENTIONAL TREATMENT

Drugs such as barbituates, anticonvulsants and sedatives.

Hydantoins are anticonvulsants given for partial seizures.

Carbamazepine or Valproic acid cause less dizziness than other seizure drugs.

Diones and suximides for absence attacks and psychomotor attacks (petit mal).

Phenacemide is an anticonvulsant for psychomotor seizures.

Tranquilizers such as benzodiazepine (valium).

Surgery—Removal of the affected brain area (only if seizures cannot be controlled by medication, area is accessible and brain function will not be impaired).

PROBLEMS ASSOCIATED WITH CONVENTIONAL TREATMENT

The only thing the drugs do is control the seizures. They do not cure the condition, and patients must stay on medication for their entire lives.

Side effects of medication can be:

Skin rash.

Ataxia (loss of coordination and jerky eye movements).

Overgrowth of gums due to loss of folic acid (hydantoin).

Dermatitis.

Dizziness.

Double vision.

Decreased white blood count.

Tremors.

Weight gain.

Temporary hair loss.

Hepatitis.

Anemia.

Irritability.

Overactivity.

Sensitivity to bright lights.

Any surgery performed is in such a delicate area that the slightest error is not reversible and the patient could be reduced to a vegetative state.

ALTERNATIVE NATURAL REMEDIES

Diet

A high protein, low carbohydrate diet is very important because it lessens the effects of the glucose derived from carbohydrates on the brain, thereby decreasing the overstimulation of electrical activity (Ketogenic diet).

Eliminate all possible allergy causing foods.

Counteract hypoglycemia (low blood sugar) by eliminating sugary foods and simple carbohydrates.

Avoid all refined foods.

Avoid eating too much at one time. Several small meals are better than fewer large ones.

Do not eat for three to four hours before bedtime.

Epileptics tend to have low thyroid function. Eat thyroid stimulating foods such as potatoes, apples, mushrooms and sesame seeds.

Avoid MSG, which contains large amounts of glutamic acid. An overabundance of glutamic acid in the brain causes seizures.

Supplements

Folic acid, 800 mcg (highest amount available), take 2 three times daily. This nutrient is depleted by seizure medication.

Vitamin B6, 100 mg. three times daily, has an anti-seizure effect. (Be aware it may lessen the effect of seizure medication.)

Magnesium citrate or aspartate, 400 mg. three times daily, for suppression of neuronal burst firing.

Manganese, 50 mg. twice daily, is helpful in controlling major and minor motor seizures.

Zinc picolinate, 30 mg. twice daily (anticonvulsants may cause a zinc deficiency).

Choline, 5 grams daily. Increase to 16 grams over a three month period. This is a precurser to aceytlcholine, a neurotransmitter which either overproduces or underproduces, leading to faulty electrical brain activity.

Dimethyl glycine, precurser of glycine (a neuroinhibitory amino acid), 125 mg. twice daily.

Vitamin E, 400 I.U. Increase to 2000 I.U. over a three month period.

Herbs

Black cohash acts as a sedative for the central nervous system.

Blue cohash has strong anti-spasmodic effects. (Avoid if pregnant.)

Lobelia is a powerful relaxant.

Mistletoe is a natural tranquilizer.

Skullcap is good for the nerves, relieves stress and aids sleep.

Amino Acids

L-Taurine, 500 mg. four times daily, on an empty stomach, is a calming neurotransmitter. It makes the cell membranes in the brain more electrically stable and prevents erratic firing.

GABA reduces neuron activity and helps decrease the likelihood of seizures.

Avoid aspartic acid and glutamic acid since these are excitory amino acids. Foods to avoid because they are high in these amino acids are ham, wild game, luncheon meats, sausage, turkey, pork, cottage cheese and wheat germ.

FIBROID TUMORS

DEFINITION

Fibroid tumors are an enlargement of the fibrous tissue in the uterus. They often bleed, and if bleeding is excessive it could cause anemia. Fibroids can also lead to a malfunction of the uterus during pregnancy. Approximately half of all women have fibroids, the majority of which are benign growths. After menopause most fibroids shrink, providing the woman does not take estrogen.

CAUSES

Pregnancy after age 35.

Overproduction of estrogen from high estrogen-producing foods.

Imbalance of estrogen and progesterone.

Overactivity of the two active types of estrogen—estrone and estradiol

Underactivity of the thyroid gland.

Overingestion of PABA and Folic acid in the diet.

CONVENTIONAL TREATMENT

Hysterectomy—The surgical removal of the uterus.

Myomectomy—The removal of the fibroids by surgery or with a laser. Most of these are done in France. Very few are performed in the United States.

Antihormone therapy to reduce estrogen—Tamoxifen, Megase, Danozol, Lupron.

PROBLEMS ASSOCIATED WITH CONVENTIONAL TREATMENT

Hysterectomy—Following a hysterectomy, your risk of a heart attack increases by a factor of three because the uterus produces prostacyclin which protects women against heart disease. Following the surgery, the vagina is shorter and therefore sexual pleasure is impaired. The pelvic bones spread, and some women have to wear a size or two larger. Muscles, ligaments and tendons are cut, causing lower back pain. The bladder will often prolapse (drop) and urinary infections become common.

Myomectomy—This procedure is not performed routinely in the United States.

Tamoxifen, Megase, Danozol and Lupron are medicines which slow production of the female hormones. When taken for long periods of time, they can cause osteoporosis, heart problems, obesity and skin problems. They can also exacerbate any condition where female hormones are needed.

ALTERNATIVE NATURAL REMEDIES

Thyroid Stimulation

Increase activity of the thyroid gland since an underactive thyroid allows overproduction of fat in the body which stimulates estrogen production.

Do some form of aerobic exercise.

Do not eat the following vegetables containing thioxazidone, which blocks the thyroid's production of its hormone, thyroxin.

Cabbage	Beets
Rutabaga	Soy beans
Spinach	Turnips

Eat the following foods which stimulate the thyroid.

Potatoes	Apples
Sesame seeds	

Take the following supplements which stimulate the thyroid. It is best to take these on an empty stomach.

Kelp, 150 mcg. (iodine) three times a day.

Tyrosine, 500 mg. four times a day.

B1 (thiamine), 100 mg. three times a day.

Diet

Too much estrogen prevents the most efficient use of oxygen in the uterus. Oxygen is necessary to prevent enlargement of the cells. Avoid the following foods containing PABA or folic acid, since these substances increase estrogen production:

Legumes	Endive
Oats	Wheat germ
Alfalfa	Brewer's yeast
Sunflower seeds	Liver

Supplements

Recommended supplements to process estrogen through the liver so it becomes a less active type of the hormone are:

B complex, 100 mg. without PABA or folic acid, once a day.

B6, 100 mg. three times a day.

Lipotropic factor, 1000 mg. (choline, inositol, and methionine) twice a day.

Vitamin E, 150 I.U. once a day.

Herbs

Red clover combination, 2 tablets three times a day and 1 silymarin (milk thistle) three times a day clears the liver of toxins so it can break down estrogens properly.

Red raspberry strengthens walls of the uterus, settles nausea and prevents hemorrhage.

Queen of the Meadow helps alleviate uterine pain, acts as a mild diuretic and an antiseptic to the system.

False unicorn corrects almost all problems of the female reproductive organs.

GALLSTONES

DEFINITION

An accumulation of crystallized cholesterol and bile that forms stones. The condition is most common in women over 40 who are overweight and have had children. It is often found in diabetics, the obese and the elderly. Approximately half the population with gallstones do not have symptoms.

Symptoms of gallstones are:

Jaundice (skin turns yellowish).

Clay colored stools.

Dark urine.

The following two symptoms usually occur within three to four hours after ingesting heavy fat or fried foods:

Severe right upper abdominal pain that may radiate to the shoulder and back.

Vomiting and/or nausea.

CAUSES

Liver dysfunction causing production of abnormal bile.

Insufficient fiber in the diet.

A deficiency in vitamin C. This vitamin helps convert cholesterol into bile acids.

CONVENTIONAL TREATMENT

Surgery—Removal of the gallbladder and/or gallstones. Newer methods recently developed remove the stones and are less invasive.

Dissolving the stones with chenodeoxycholic acid (found in goose liver and goose bile).

PROBLEMS ASSOCIATED WITH CONVENTIONAL TREATMENT

Scar tissue from surgery attracts bacteria and fungi to the area. The bacteria and fungi then attack the surrounding tissue causing it to become inflamed and leading to further deterioration in the area.

Removing the gall bladder does not address the situation which caused the stones in the first place. The problem originates in the liver, which is dysfunctional and producing abnormal cholesterol and bile.

Drug therapy may cause diarrhea and an increase in serum cholesterol.

ALTERNATIVE NATURAL REMEDIES

Diet

Strict elimination of highly saturated and cholesterol laden foods such as high fat dairy products, meat products, fried or scrambled eggs and oils.

Avoid sugar and sugar-laden foods.

The possibility of insufficient digestive acids and enzymes should be addressed since these determine the overall breakdown of ingested foods.

Production of cholesterol does not come just from ingesting it in the foods consumed. Even vegetarians can have high cholesterol if they are under stress. Cholesterol is a component of adrenalin. During periods of stress the liver overproduces cholesterol in its effort to aid the adrenal glands in their manufacture of adrenalin. Overall body cholesterol rises, and if the process continues over a long period of time, the liver will break down and eventually become dysfunctional.

High fiber type foods absorb and eliminate cholesterol and bile by keeping them soluble and slowing or stopping their absorption by the body. A high bile content in the colon is a leading cause of colon cancer.

Foods with a high fiber content include:

Legumes.
Bran.
Whole grains.
Brown rice.
Psyllium seeds.
Whole grain pasta and spaghetti.

Other types of fiber useful in removing cholesterol and bile acids are:

Guar gum.
Apple pectin.
Lignin.

Oat bran.

Wheat bran.

Supplements

Lecithin, 1200 mg. capsules six times daily or three tablespoons of the granular form, is useful to eliminate and break down fats. It is also found in soy beans and eggs (soft cooked or poached only since lecithin is destroyed by oxidation at high temperatures used in frying).

Multiple digestive enzymes, 1 or 2 with each meal.

Aloe vera gel, 2 tbsp. three times daily. Helps entire digestive tract. (Store in refrigerator.)

Acidophilus, enteric coated, 2 billion cells each capsule, four times daily on empty stomach.

Multi-vitamin and mineral, one daily.

Vitamin C, 500 mg. four times daily.

Fish oil, 180 mg. EPA, 8 capsules daily breaks up gallstones.

Herbs

Buckthorn breaks bile down into its normal component parts.

Hydrangea prevents gravel deposits. (Gallstones are gravel.)

Parsley is good for all liver problems.

Silymarin (milk thistle) rebuilds liver cells.

Cascara sagrada helps the body rid itself of gallstones.

Amino Acids

L-Methionine is a precurser of choline, and prevents fat cohesion in the liver.

L-Carnitine, 250 mg. twice daily, breaks down excess fat, lessening production of bile.

L-Taurine, 500 mg. three times daily, moderates cholesterol production and fat metabolism.

L-Threonine is essential for fat metabolism in the liver. Take according to directions on label.

Adjunctive Therapy

Castor oil packs. Soak a piece of white flannel in warm castor oil, wring it out and place over the inflamed area. Cover with plastic and apply a heating pad. Do this twice a day for one hour each sitting.

Gall bladder flush to remove stones. Do not eat anything after noon. At 7 p.m. take 4 tablespoons of olive oil followed by 2 tablespoons of fresh lemon juice. Repeat every 15 minutes until 8:45. You will have used 16 ounces of olive oil and the juice of 12 lemons.

Go to bed at 10 p.m. and lie on right side. The following morning a bowel movement should flush out the stones if they are not extremely large. The bile duct expands and is also lubricated by the oil. The stones in the duct dislodge and move into the intestines and out of the body with the bowel movement. Several movements may occur for the following two days.

GLAUCOMA

DEFINITION

A disease of the eye characterized by increased intra-ocular pressure and hardening of the surface of the eye. It is the second leading cause of blindness. Symptoms include halos around lights, impaired vision, pain, discomfort, loss of peripheral vision and the inability to adjust from light to dark areas. Early diagnosis is critical and can be done easily and painlessly by a routine eye examination.

CAUSES

Aging process, infection, genetic predisposition, tumors, trauma, hormone disorders, nutritional problems, stress and allergy. Adrenal exhaustion can cause the exacerbation of the disease.

CONVENTIONAL TREATMENT

Prescription eyedrops which improve the outflow of fluid from the eye.

Epinephrine compound which decreases production of intra-ocular fluid.

Surgery.

Laser treatments.

PROBLEMS ASSOCIATED WITH CONVENTIONAL TREATMENT

Some eyedrops cause an increased sensitivity to light, and they may cause an excessive flow of tears.

Side effects of medication can damage the heart and may lead to diabetes.

Surgery and laser treatments are performed in a delicate area and must be done by a highly qualified eye surgeon. Each case is different and more than one opinion should be sought.

ALTERNATIVE NATURAL REMEDIES

Diet

Eat foods high in vitamin C such as vegetables and fruits.

Foods good for weak eyes are watercress, carrots, onion, broccoli and cabbage.

Drink fluids in small amounts at a time since excess fluid intake raises eye pressure.

Avoid caffeine in all forms, including coffee, tea, chocolate and cola. Caffeine is a vasoconstrictor and raises eye pressure.

Supplements

Vitamin C (Ester C) to bowel tolerance. When diarrhea occurs, cut back dosage until normal bowel function returns and remain at that dosage.

Vitamin A, Beta carotene, 25,000 I.U. twice daily.

Vitamin A, Fish liver oil, 25,000 I.U. once daily.

Vitamin D, 400 I.U. once daily (works with Vitamin A for healthy eyes).

Vitamin B2 (Riboflavin) is important for healthy eyes.

Vitamin B5, Pantothene, 300 mg. three times daily.

Vitamin B1, 200 mg. twice daily.

Manganese, 50 mg. twice daily.

Choline, 650 mg. twice daily.

Quercetin (bioflavanoid) 500 mg. three times daily.

Herbs

Eyebright strengthens all parts of the eye and provides elasticity to the nerves and optic devices responsible for sight.

Golden seal is a natural antibiotic for eye problems.

Bilberry aids in vision problems. A jam made from this herb was used by pilots in World War II for more effective night vision.

Amino Acids

L-Glutathione, 250 mg. twice daily, prevents oxidation of cellular membrane of the cornea.

Adjunctive Therapy

Palming—Close eyes as tight as possible without straining. Place cupped palms over eyes so there is total darkness. Energy circulating through the body into the arms and hands revitalizes diseased cells in the eyes. Do this for five minutes once daily.

Sunning—With closed eyes face the sun in early morning, before 9 a.m. Start with 15 seconds and add 15 seconds daily until reaching 5 minutes. Then go into a shaded area and rest with closed eyes for 2 minutes.

Spheno Palatine Block opens circulation in the eye by blocking the autonomic nervous system. (Must be done by a Holistic Medical Doctor.)

GOUT

DEFINITION

A disease characterized by swelling, pain and inflammation in the joints. A high uric acid content in the blood leaves deposits of uric acid crystals in and around the tissues of the joints in the extremities, especially the big toe. Gout usually occurs in males. High uric acid levels are often seen in those with high intellectual achievement, high intelligence, the overachievers and high aspirers.

CAUSES

High uric acid levels occur from the inability to metabolize proteins from purine type foods. Uric acid crystals form in the joints causing the body to release harmful chemicals that cause inflammation and severe pain in the affected areas. Poor diet, age, diuretic type medication and overweight predisposes the susceptibility to gout.

CONVENTIONAL TREATMENT

Anti-inflammatory drugs.

Colchicine from the root of meadow saffron. It works by decreasing amounts of harmful chemicals the body produces in response to the crystals formed in the joints rather than by lowering amounts of uric acid in the body.

Medications to lower uric acid levels and promote excretion through the kidneys.

Medications to prevent the formation of uric acid stones.

PROBLEMS ASSOCIATED WITH CONVENTIONAL TREATMENT

Anti-inflammatories can cause dizziness, nausea, headache, constipation, diarrhea, vomiting, internal bleeding and decreased urinary output.

Colchicine can cause numbness in the hands and feet, fever, abdominal pain, nausea, vomiting, weakness, hair loss, and abnormal bleeding or bruising.

Drugs to lower uric acid levels and prevent stones may weaken kidney function due to the over-excretion of uric acid through the kidneys, and may force your kidneys to work too hard.

ALTERNATIVE NATURAL REMEDIES

Diet

Eliminate all purine type foods such as:

Organ meats, anchovies, sardines, shrimp, gravies, fried foods, cream, ice cream, pastries, rich desserts, alcohol, spices and mushrooms.

Avoid caffeine since it impairs kidney function which is needed to get uric acid out of the system.

Potassium rich foods protect against gout. Use more vegetable juices, leafy green vegetables, legumes, potatoes and fish.

Sour cherries and strawberries help inflammation and pain at the onset of the disease by getting uric acid out of your body and they also alkalize the system. For greatest effectiveness, consume them between meals.

Grapes are high in alkalines which lessen the acidity of uric acid and aid in its elimination from the body.

Parsley acts as a natural diuretic.

Pears relieve inflammation of the kidneys.

The diet should consist mainly of natural organic foods. Use nuts, seeds, whole grains such as brown rice, millet, buckwheat, quinoa (pronounced keenwa) and corn. Other helpful foods are beans and complex carbohydrate vegetables that grow underground, including potatoes, beets, yams and carrots.

A high fiber diet also aids in eliminating uric acid by absorbing bile acids formed in the liver. These bile acids can act as a precursor to uric acid.

Supplements

High Vitamin C (Ester C), to bowel tolerance (when diarrhea occurs). Then cut back amount until normal bowel function returns.

Vitamin B5 Pantothene, 300 mg. three times daily, as an anti-inflammatory.

Folic acid, two 800 mcg. tablets three times daily.

Bromelin, 500 mg. twice daily as an anti-inflammatory.

Fish oil, two 1000 mg. capsules three times daily.

Magnesium citrate, 400 mg. three times daily, as an anti-spasmodic to relieve pain.

Herbs

Black cohash moderates blood acidity.

Saffron neutralizes uric acid buildup.

Devil's claw is a natural cleansing agent for toxic impurities.

Nettle contains alkaloids which neutralize uric acid.

Hydrangea is an anti-inflammatory.

Amino Acids

L-Glycine, 500 mg. four times daily between meals, acts as an anti-acid.

L-Glutathione,100 mg. twice daily on empty stomach, increases renal cleansing of uric acid.

L-Glutamine, 500 mg. four times daily on empty stomach, is an antacid.

L-Methionine, 250 mg. twice daily on empty stomach, detoxifies purines.

DLPA Phenylalanine, 500 mg. four times daily on empty stomach, decreases pain.

Adjunctive Therapies

Bicarbonate of soda helps alkalize the system. Take 1/2 teaspoon in water twice daily.

Castor oil packs. Soak a piece of white flannel in warm castor oil, wring it out and place over the inflamed area. Cover with plastic and apply a heating pad. Do this twice a day for one hour each sitting.

Fasting—If possible, no food for three to four days. Drink distilled water and five to six glasses of green vegetable juices or apple juice daily.

Headaches

DEFINITION

Pain and pressure in different areas of the head. Headaches are not a disease. They are a symptom of an underlying condition.

Sinus headaches are due to the overproduction of mucous in the membranes.

Vascular headaches are caused by the tightening and contraction of muscles in the area of the neck, forehead and scalp.

Migraine headaches are caused by the alternating constriction and dilation of blood vessels in the brain. The common migraine is accompanied by an uneasy feeling, nausea, depression and tingling in the arms and legs. The classic migraine is preceded by visual disturbances such as flashing lights, sensitivity to noise, weakness and dizziness.

CAUSES

Nutrient deficiencies.

Bruxism (grinding of teeth).

TMJ misalignment.

Food allergies.

Side effect of medication.

Electrical imbalance of ions in atmospheric oxygen.

Caffeine withdrawal.

Lack of sleep.

Premenstrual syndrome.

Birth control pills.

MSG.

Hunger.

Constipation.

Food additives (preservatives and chemicals).

Alcohol.

Air pollution.

Bacterial and Viral infections.

Eye problems and improper eyeglasses.

Tension.

Hypoglycemia (low blood sugar).

Overexposure to sun.

Dehydration.

Overproduction of carbon dioxide and reduction of oxygen supply which can be caused by sleeping with covers pulled over the head.

Deficiency in red blood cell choline levels.

Migraine headaches can be activated by tyramine type foods such as aged cheese, nuts, shell fish, pork, bananas and wine.

CONVENTIONAL TREATMENT

Painkillers.

Anti-depressants.

Ergotamine.

Methysergide for prevention of migraine headaches.

PROBLEMS ASSOCIATED WITH CONVENTIONAL TREATMENT

Strong painkillers can be addictive. Analgesics such as aspirin can cause bleeding from the stomach. Phanacetin can lead to chronic kidney disease.

Anti-depressants may cause drowsiness, blurred vision, nervousness and weight gain.

Ergotamine is used to constrict blood vessels in the scalp and decreases their pulsation. Its side effect can be destruction of the arteries in your limbs, eyes or heart.

Methysergide may lead to fibroid growth in the kidneys.

ALTERNATIVE NATURAL REMEDIES

Diet

Eliminate alcohol, cold foods, ice cream, ice cubes, frozen desserts and tyramine type foods such as aged cheese, nuts, shell fish, pork, bananas and wine.

Avoid chocolate, tea, cola drinks and coffee since all contain caffeine.

Avoid dairy products.

Avoid citrus fruits which may precipitate a migraine attack.

Check food labels for MSG, additives and preservatives.

Beware of salad bars. Check to be sure that sulfites have not been used to keep vegetables appearing fresh.

Migraine headaches are basically an acid condition. Try to keep the system more alkaline by eating raw fruits, vegetables and sprouts. Do not eat acid producing foods such as whole grains, sugars and food from animal sources until headache diminishes. Carrot and celery juice help relieve migraine headaches.

Supplements

Niacin, 100 mg. three times daily. Increase slowly until taking 300 mg. three times daily. High dosages sometimes cause flushing. It is no cause for alarm and usually disappears in 30 minutes.

Vitamin B complex, 50 mg. twice daily for stress.

Magnesium citrate, 400 mg. three times daily for pain relief.

Vitamin E, 400 I.U. twice daily (work up to this dose slowly), aids circulation by thinning the blood.

Fish oil, 1000 mg. two capsules three times daily.

Vitamin C (Ester C) 1000 mg. three times daily, inhibits platelet aggregation (clumping) preventing the release of excessive levels of arachidonic acid.

Oxygen therapy using the following:

CoEnzyme Q10, 30 mg. three times daily.

Dimethyl glycine, 125 mg. twice daily.

Germanium, 100 mg. three times daily.

Herbs

Feverfew alleviates pain of migraine headaches because it makes you less responsive to the chemicals that cause spasms in the muscles surrounding your brain. Do not take more than 14 consecutive days as it becomes ineffective after that time.

Basil draws poisons out of the body.

Blessed thistle aids circulation and helps oxygenate the brain.

Ephedra acts as a vasodilator.

Ginger removes congestion.

Peppermint allows oxygen into the bloodstream.

White willow bark has an effect similar to aspirin.

Thyme has been used for centuries in the treatment of headaches.

Amino Acids

DLPA Phenylalanine, 500 mg. four times daily on empty stomach, decreases pain.

GABA, 500 mg. twice daily on empty stomach, is a muscle relaxant.

Adjunctive Remedies

Hydrogen peroxide gel 35 percent, rubbed into soles of feet once daily.

Relaxation techniques such as meditation, biofeedback and imagery.

Daily aerobic exercise to strengthen and enhance lung capacity for oxygen intake.

Allergy testing for food and environmental factors.

A four day fast (taking liquids only) allows most toxins to be eliminated from the body, which will lessen inflammatory processes in the head.

HEART DISEASE
(CORONARY OCCLUSIONS)

DEFINITION

The breakdown of the function of the heart leading to an inability to provide the body with blood, its life-giving force. Heart muscle deteriorates to the degree that its pumping action is impeded. This failure in the heart muscle is due mainly to a lack of oxygen and nutrients, which are carried to it by the coronary arteries. Deposits from the blood, such as cholesterol, triglycerides, fibrinogens, proteins, calcium and platelets clumping together, clog these arteries which feed the heart. This impedes the continuous flow of blood to the heart muscle.

Risk factors are elevated cholesterol and triglyceride levels, high blood pressure, diabetes, obesity, smoking, lack of exercise, high uric acid levels, genetics and stress. Club fingers and creased ear lobes are visual indicators of possible future heart problems. Most of these factors can be controlled by an altered lifestyle. Forty percent of people who have heart attacks have no risk factors, and 250,000 people a year have painless (silent) heart attacks.

CAUSES

The primary cause of occlusion to the coronary arteries is arteriosclerosis (hardening of the arteries) and atherosclerosis (clogging of the arteries).

Homogenized milk can be destructive to the interior surface of the arteries. Xanthine oxidase, an enzyme in homogenized milk, may have the ability to irritate the inner surface of the arteries, which could be the cause of the initial crack in the arterial wall. These cracks must then be sealed by cholesterol, platelets, triglycerides, fibrinogens and calcium which then cause clots and blockage. In addition, the fat molecules in homogenized milk are reduced to microscopic size and are able to get into the bloodstream quickly.

The coronary arteries can go into spasm if there is a deficiency of magnesium in the blood.

A deficiency of Vitamin B6 which is needed to break down the methionine in organ meats to a less destructive compound. If methionine is not broken down properly, it causes irritations in the vessels and arteriosclerosis is initiated.

Too much insulin in the blood weakens the heart because it encourages growth of the epithelium cells that line the blood vessels, stimulates the sympathetic nervous system leading to an increased heart rate and causes sodium retention which increases blood pressure.

Eye drops used for the treatment of glaucoma can make heart failure much worse.

Undue stress can cause the adrenal glands to overproduce adrenalin, which increases the heart rate to such a degree that a heart attack could be precipitated.

Low levels of Vitamin E, which are more of a factor in heart disease than high cholesterol or high blood pressure.

CONVENTIONAL TREATMENT

Medications and surgery such as:

Diuretics reduce the amount of fluid in the system in order to relieve pressure on the heart.

A.C.E. inhibits adrenalin.

Calcium channel blockers hold back calcium from the heart muscle, preventing too strong a heart contraction.

Beta blockers interfere with the nerves' beta fibers, lowering the sympathetic nervous function, which is needed to decrease the susceptibility to stress and nervousness.

Nitroglycerine improves the supply of blood and oxygen to the heart, relieves angina pain and aids in prevention of heart attacks.

Procainamide restores a regular heart beat and slows down an overactive heart.

Blood thinners such as coumadin.

Aspirin as a blood thinner.

Cholesterol lowering drugs.

Low fat diet.

Coronary bypass surgery which is the bypassing of the blocked artery or arteries that feed the heart muscle.

Heart replacement, either with a donor heart or a synthetic heart.

Angioplasty is the insertion of a catheter, with a balloon attached, into the blocked area of the artery. The balloon is expanded, pushing the blockage toward the walls of the artery, allowing blood to flow freely and fully.

Angiograms for diagnostic purposes.

Antibiotics for those with mitral valve prolapse, before having dental work, to prevent endocarditis.

PROBLEMS ASSOCIATED WITH CONVENTIONAL TREATMENT

Angiograms show a two dimensional view, but blood flow in the artery is three dimensional. Therefore the angiogram does not give the full picture of true coronary action. In addition, dye that is injected produces vasoconstriction (spasms) which can cause a heart attack.

Medications are just blocking agents, merely address symptoms, rather than causes, and have side effects.

Diuretics given to lower blood pressure cause overproduction of urine which leads to the loss of other electrolytes such as calcium, magnesium, sodium and potassium.

A.C.E. used to inhibit adrenalin production may at times act in a negative way in situations where the body needs an extra boost of energy (for the fight or flight response) and it is not available.

Calcium channel blockers and beta blockers often slow your heart to such a degree that it cuts down its strength to supply your body with its necessary energy.

Nitroglycerine can cause headaches, skin rashes, flushing, nausea and dizziness.

Procainamide may cause diarrhea, vomiting, joint pain, fever and depression.

Coumadin was originally used as rat poison. The rodent's blood became so thin that severe internal bleeding lead to its death. Patients on this drug must be monitored constantly to be sure their blood does not become so thin that they could bleed to death.

Aspirin destroys stomach tissues and may cause ulcerative conditions in the stomach.

A prominent heart surgeon has speculated that most of the patients operated on had either normal or below normal cholesterol levels.

During bypass surgery a vein is taken from the thigh to bypass an artery in the heart. Veins are not designed for this purpose since they are narrower and not as strong as arteries. Eventually the vein can break down if the diet is not changed and plaque accumulation causes another blockage. When this procedure is performed, the heart has to be stopped, but the blood supply to the body must continue. A mechanical device (heart-lung machine) is used to shunt blood from the body, through the machine and back. As blood flows through the metal parts of the machine, it picks up metal ions and transfers them into the body. These ions are heavy metals which are toxic to the system, especially the brain, and can cause loss of memory, slowdown of cognitive thought processes and spaciness. Although these side effects are usually temporary, some patients have them for years.

During bypass surgery, the death rate is at least two percent. Some statistics say six percent. Five percent have immediate heart attacks. Five percent have immediate strokes. Twenty percent have mental disturbances.

Angioplasty has failed to live up to its expectations. By removing plaque formation, it may be possible that pieces of plaque can loosen and continue along in the bloodstream, possibly causing embolisms in other parts of the body.

Patients with mitral valve prolapse, who do not have a murmur or thickening of the valve, are not candidates for endocarditis and do not need antibiotics before going to the dentist.

ALTERNATIVE NATURAL REMEDIES

Diet

Address obesity. If overweight, the patient must lose weight by reducing the fat content of the diet. Body fat is made from sugars and high fat animal foods. The best type diet for weight loss is a high protein, low-fat, low carbohydrate diet. Many carbohydrates convert to sugar (glucose) in the body. Foods to avoid are processed foods, high sugar content foods, junk foods, and alcohol. In some cases (diabetes), fruits, grains and starchy vegetables must also be avoided. The diet should consist of salads, greens, fish, low-fat organic chicken and turkey, lean organic lamb, veal, pork, non-fat cottage cheese, Swiss cheese and yogurt. Soft boiled or poached eggs are allowed since they do not raise cholesterol when cooked at these lower temperatures. Lecithin in eggs helps lower cholesterol.

Dietary cholesterol is found only in animal type foods and not in foods grown in the field. If not overweight, eat the following high fiber foods to lower cholesterol: whole grains, brown rice, nuts, seeds, fruits with skin, starchy vegetables with the skins such as beets, yams, carrots and corn.

Avoid margarine. It melts at 114 degrees. The body is only 98 degrees. Therefore it is not broken down and leaves a residue which can cause clogging of the arteries.

Weight loss is a more important factor than lowering cholesterol to avoid straining the heart.

Supplements

Heart function enhancers:

Vitamin C (Ester C) 1000 mg. four times daily, helps reduce free radical production in the heart muscle.

Vitamin A, fish liver oil, 25,000 I.U. once daily and

Vitamin A, Beta carotene, 25,000 I.U. twice daily, stimulate the immune system.

Vitamin E, 200 I.U. daily, then build up slowly to 1000 I.U. Latest studies show a low Vitamin E content in the blood leads to more heart attacks than high cholesterol readings. Chlorine in drinking water destroys Vitamin E.

Magnesium citrate, 400 mg. three times daily, decreases the susceptibility of coronary artery spasms.

Calcium citrate, 400 mg. twice daily, strengthens the heart muscle.

Potassium, 99 mg. five times daily, acts as a heart relaxant. Deficiencies are rare since it is found in abundance in fruits, vegetables, beans, nuts, seeds and grains. If enough of the foods are consumed, supplements are not necessary.

Copper supplementation may be necessary since low red blood cell levels of this mineral can have a deleterious effect on the heart. However, we do not suggest copper supplements unless levels are checked, since some individuals may have too high a level of copper in their system. It would be better to increase consumption of liver (not if cholesterol is high), whole grains, beans, green leafy vegetables, fish and almonds.

CoEnzyme Q10, 30 mg. three times daily, helps prevent further damage after heart attack caused by lack of oxygen.

L-Carnitine (amino acid), 250 mg. three times daily, strengthens the heart muscle by utilizing energy in the cells in the wall of the heart muscle.

Cholesterol lowering supplements:

Lecithin, 1200 mg. six times daily, or 3 tbsp. of granules daily, emulsifies fat.

Fish oil, 1000 mg. capsules six times daily.

Garlic (enteric coated), 500 mg. four times daily.

Chromium picolinate, 200 mcg. three times daily.

Psyllium seed husks, 1 tbsp. in a glass of water morning and evening. This is not necessary if enough high fiber foods such as brown rice, nuts, seeds, fruits with skins and starchy vegetables, including potatoes, beets, yams, carrots and corn are consumed. Take only if cutting back on these foods for the purpose of weight loss.

Pantothene, 300 mg. three times daily.

Guar gum, per label.

GLA in the form of Evening primrose oil, or borage oil, per label.

CoEnzyme Q10, 30 mg. twice daily.

Blood thinning supplements:

Garlic (enteric coated), 500 mg. four times daily.

Fish oil, 1000 mg. six times daily.

Vitamin E, start with 200 I.U. and build slowly to 1000 I.U. to avoid increasing blood pressure.

Lecithin, 1200 mg. six times daily or 3 tbsp. of granules daily.

Herbs

Hawthorne, in tea or capsule form, per label, strengthens the heart muscle.

Amino Acids

L-Taurine, 500 mg. four times daily on empty stomach, moderates cholesterol production, prevents cardiac loss of potassium and removes fluid from the body, decreasing the overload on the heart.

L-Glutamine, 500 mg. four times daily on an empty stomach, cuts down on the loss of potassium, sodium and electrolytes.

L-Histidine, per directions on label, is a powerful vasodilator.

Note: Some of these supplements may be listed in more than one category. Do not take double doses!

Non-Invasive Diagnostic Tests

RNCA (radioactive nuclear cyni angiogram). This is done by means of injection of a radioactive isotope. It delivers half the radiation of a chest X-ray.

Thalium stress test.

MUGA (multiple gated pool) ejection test.

First pass study.

Digital subtraction angiogram (uses dye instead of a catheter). The picture looks exactly like an angiogram.

Exercise

Collateral arterial circulation is increased by exercise. This is the body's natural way to protect the heart. If a coronary artery becomes blocked, these arteries can bypass the blockage site. Aerobic type exercise strengthens the heart muscle and allows it to operate more efficiently. Anaerobic exercise, such as weight lifting or resistance training, is not good for a weak heart because it raises blood pressure too much.

Placebo Effect

There have been reports of patients where bypass surgery was started, but not completed. The patients awakened with an incision on the chest, thought the surgery had been performed and reported feeling better.

Hemorrhoids

DEFINITION

Hemorrhoids are ruptured distended veins located in the anal area. Previously, they were called piles. Sometimes they itch or bleed and can cause severe pain or discomfort. Hemorrhoids are similar to any type of varicosity in the body in that they are a weakening of the membrane of the cell leading to leakage of cellular fluids and swelling of the veins.

CAUSES

Constipation.

Diarrhea.

Straining while moving the bowels.

Obesity.

Pregnancy.

Heavy lifting.

Sedentary life.

Improper diet.

Prolonged sitting or standing.

CONVENTIONAL TREATMENT

Surgery—Hemorrhoidectomy, the removal of the swollen veins.

Rubber banding (ligation).

Injections to shrink the swollen veins.

Mineral oil taken orally to lubricate and soften stools.

Over the counter analgesics and ointments for shrinkage.

PROBLEMS ASSOCIATED WITH CONVENTIONAL TREATMENT

Scar tissue that forms after surgery can—later in life—cause more problems than the original hemorrhoids.

Side effects of surgery are weakening of your immune system, and the possibility of contracting other diseases or infections in the hospital.

Other methods merely address symptoms rather than causes, and the problem usually recurs unless changes are made in the diet and lifestyle.

Mineral oil coats the sides of the intestines, slowing absorption of vitamins A, D, E and K which are all vital nutrients.

ALTERNATIVE NATURAL REMEDIES

Diet

A high fiber diet is essential for digested material to have enough bulk to exert pressure on the interior lining of the colon to signal that a bowel movement is necessary. Fiber enhances the absorption of fluid into the feces giving them a soft consistency which allows an easy evacuation.

Recommended foods are bran, whole grains, fruit with skins, green salads and green vegetables. Also include starchy vegetables with skins such as beans, peas, lentils, potatoes, yams, carrots, beets and corn.

Drink at least 8 to 10 glasses of water daily to enhance absorption of fluid into the stool for softening purposes.

In extreme cases of constipation or diarrhea, add psyllium seed husks to the diet one to three times daily. They act as a bulking agent and normalize bowel function. It is important to take sufficient fluid when using this method. After mixing the material according to directions, be sure to drink an extra glass of water, otherwise it will have the opposite effect.

Diarrhea can cause as many problems with hemorrhoids as constipation. Constant bowel movements can inflame the area and lead to other anal problems such as fissures (cracks) which become infected, and fistulas (abnormal ducts or passages). Diarrhea is caused by undigested material that reaches the colon, causing inflammation and signaling the brain that a bowel movement is necessary. If food is not properly metabolized it acts as a foreign body and is attacked by antibodies, causing inflammation. The inflammatory process may cause chronic diarrhea.

Eliminate highly sugared foods and those contaminated with chemicals and pesticides. These ingredients stress the body and cause an overreaction that tightens all organs, muscles and glands, disturbing metabolism to such a degree that undigested material is allowed to reach the colon.

If sensitivity to a food, such as a particular grain or dairy products, is causing diarrhea, it is best to eliminate it or just ingest it every fourth day in order not to overtax the digestive system. A person can be sensitive to a particular food without actually suffering from an allergy to it.

Supplements

Rutin (bioflavanoid), 200 mg. three times daily, strengthens cell membrane of your anal veins to prevent leakage.

Vitamin K, per directions on label, to clot bleeding hemorrhoids.

Vitamin A, Beta carotene, 25,000 I.U. twice daily.

Vitamin E, 400 I.U. twice daily. Work up to this amount slowly.

VM75 multi-vitamin/mineral, 1 daily.

Vitamin C (Ester C), 2000 mg. four times daily.

Acidophilus, enteric coated, 2 billion plus viable cells each capsule, three times daily on empty stomach.

Intestinal Clay, per label, attracts toxins which are then eliminated.

Herbs

Aloe vera gel, 2 ounces, three times daily, cleans, soothes and heals hemorrhoids, plus reduces chance of infection and scarring.

Myrrh is a powerful antiseptic for mucous membranes, helps soothe inflammation in colon and speeds the healing process.

White oak bark helps heal damaged tissues in your anus and is an intestinal tonic for diarrhea.

Amino Acids

L-Glutamine, 500 mg. on empty stomach twice daily, promotes regeneration of intestinal mucosa.

L-Arginine, 1000 mg. three times daily on empty stomach, promotes wound healing.

Adjunctive Treatments

Apply vitamin E oil topically after every bowel movement. The oil can be purchased in health food stores or you can puncture a capsule with a needle and squeeze out the contents.

Be sure the anal area is thoroughly cleansed. Moisten toilet paper.

Aloe vera gel can be applied topically.

Shape a slice of peeled potato or a large clove of garlic into a suppository and insert into your anus. These act as a local antibiotic if the area is infected.

Sitz baths are soothing.

Acidophilus yogurt applied to area relieves itching.

Malt syrup extract taken orally relieves itching.

Walking strengthens muscles, ligaments and tendons.

Do abdominal exercises to strengthen muscles in the area that aid normal activity of colon.

Colonics, performed by a licensed therapist, are a system of cleansing the colon with a special machine. A continuous flow of water is infused into the colon, cleaning accumulated debris from its interior surface. This debris can remain collected on the sides of the colon for years and builds up to such a degree that it interferes with the amount of fluid which is reabsorbed back into the system through the wall of the colon. Retained debris can also lead to absorption of toxins.

HERPES (GENITAL)

DEFINITION

A viral disease related to the chicken pox virus. It lies dormant in the body until the immune system is weakened from factors such as medications, emotional and physical stress, smoking, recreational drugs, alcohol and sugar. The immune system has lost its ability to protect the body against overactivity of this particular virus. Once in the body, the virus never leaves and can only be kept under control by maintaining a strong immune system. Severe cases can lead to brain and eye damage.

CAUSES

Sexual contact, either intercourse or oral.

Kissing.

Newborns can contract the disease from the cervix or vagina during delivery. For the baby's protection, a cesarean section might be indicated.

CONVENTIONAL TREATMENT

Medication such as acyclovir.

Topical ointments containing providone (iodine solution).

Lithium cream.

Ice.

PROBLEMS ASSOCIATED WITH CONVENTIONAL TREATMENT

Sometimes when the medication is stopped a more serious outbreak may occur.

Medication depletes the immune system and, in my opinion, is not the proper therapy for this type disease. Enhancing rather than depressing the immune system leads to a faster long-term remission. At its optimal level, the immune system would destroy the herpes virus and diminish the disease quickly.

ALTERNATIVE NATURAL REMEDIES

Diet

Stimulate the immune system by excluding all known allergic type foods or other immune depressants such as chemicals, preservatives and sugars.

Avoid foods containing the amino acid L-Argenine which suppresses L-Lysine, the amino acid that retards growth of the herpes virus. These foods include soybeans, nuts, peanuts, turkey, pheasant, chocolate, goose and pork.

Shitake mushrooms and Reishi mushrooms enhance the immune system.

Supplements

Vitamin C (Ester C), 2000 mg. four times daily, acts as an anti-viral.

B complex, 100 mg. twice daily, for stress.

Vitamin E, work up to 800 I.U. daily.

Zinc picolinate, 50 mg. twice daily. Use this amount only during an outbreak because high amounts of zinc deplete the body of copper. When taking this much zinc, take a copper supplement, 2 to 4 mg. once daily. Depletion of copper can lead to the lowering of HDL cholesterol (the good kind).

Multi-mineral, once daily.

Vitamin A Beta carotene, 25,000 I.U. twice daily.

Vitamin A, fish liver oil, 25,000 once daily.

Monolauren, per label, acts as an anti-viral.

BHT (Butylated hydroxy toluene), 250 mg. four times daily, is a synthetic antioxidant. Do not take on empty stomach as irritation can occur.

AMP (Adenosine monophosphate) given by injection by holistic physician.

Garlic, enteric coated, 500 mg. four times daily.

Cartilade (shark cartilage), 12 per day for three weeks, acts as an anti-inflammatory.

Herbs

Myrrh is an antiseptic for the mucous membranes and can also be used as a healing antiseptic salve.

Slippery elm bark helps your adrenal glands' production of cortin, a hormone needed to fight inflammation.

Amino Acid

L-Lysine, 500 mg. four times daily on empty stomach, at outbreak. For maintenance take one capsule daily.

Adjunctive Methods

Aloe Vera used externally.

Black walnut salve used externally.

Buttermilk and yogurt applied externally eases pain and aids healing.

Hiatal Hernia

DEFINITION

An opening in the diaphragm that causes a protrusion of the upper part of the stomach into the esophagus.

CAUSES

Acids leak back into the lower part of the esophagus, causing burning and inflammation (reflux).

CONVENTIONAL TREATMENT

Antacids.

Weight loss.

Elimination of coffee, tea, chocolate and cola.

Eating several small meals rather than three large ones.

Surgery.

PROBLEMS ASSOCIATED WITH CONVENTIONAL TREATMENT

Antacids deplete hydrochloric acid in the stomach, leading to its inability to break food down to its tiniest molecule and interfering with its ability to metabolize food into necessary nutrients. They also contain aluminum which causes leaching of calcium from the bones.

Surgery causes scar tissue which attracts bacteria and fungi to the area. The bacteria and fungi then attack tissue, causing it to become inflamed and leading to further deterioration in the area.

ALTERNATIVE NATURAL REMEDIES

Diet

Do not consume large amounts of food at one time. Several small meals are better. Do not eat for at least three hours before bedtime, and never lie down right after eating.

Avoid coffee, chocolate, cola and tea which all weaken the esophageal sphincter.

Avoid acidic foods such as lemons, grapefruit, oranges and tomato juice.

Avoid spicy foods.

Eat slowly and in a peaceful atmosphere.

Do not consume liquids while eating. They dilute stomach acids and enzymes.

Refrain from ice cold drinks which can cause the stomach to contract, lessening its production of the digestive enzymes needed to break down food.

Supplements

Aloe vera gel, 2 ounces three times daily, is very soothing and healing to the entire digestive tract (keep in refrigerator).

Acidophilus, 2 billion viable cells, three times daily on empty stomach.

Multiple digestive enzymes (pancreatin), 1 or 2 with each meal. Do not take digestive enzymes containing hydrochloric acid.

Chlorophyll, per label.

VM75, multi-vitamin/mineral, 1 a day.

Charcoal pills, per label, to absorb excess gas.

Adjunctive Methods

Raise the head of the bed three inches.

Men should wear suspenders rather than tight belts to hold up their pants.

Women should not wear tight girdles or anything tight around the waist. Be sure the elastic at the top of panty hose is not too tight.

Be careful not to swallow air.

Women on hormone replacement therapy should be aware that estrogen can aggravate heartburn.

Hyperactivity

DEFINITION

A malfunction of the mechanism in the central nervous system which causes an excessive amount of energy. This high energy level leads to aggressive behavior, frustrations, poor concentration, clumsiness and poor sleeping patterns. Children with this condition suffer from poor muscle coordination, a short attention span and are easily distracted. They often get low grades in school even though they may have high intelligence. Another name for this condition is minimal brain dysfunction syndrome or attention defect disorder (ADD).

CAUSES

Allergies to foods, chemicals and environmental pollutants.

Foods with a high sugar content may lead to hyperactivity.

Coloring agents used in processed foods.

Preservatives used in processed foods

Foods containing salicylates such as peaches, plums, prunes, apricots, apples, cherries, grapes, tomatoes, mint, almonds, cucumbers, pickles, oranges, strawberries and raspberries.

Caffeine, found in chocolate or any type beverage such as coffee, tea, cola and other sodas.

CONVENTIONAL TREATMENT

Drugs to lower hyperactivity such as Ritalin.

Drugs to increase attention span.

PROBLEMS ASSOCIATED WITH CONVENTIONAL TREATMENT

Drugs address symptoms rather than causes. The child may be allergic to coloring agents and binders in the medication, and may actually become more hyperactive when taking it. In order to be effective, the amount of medication taken may lead to lethargy or inactivity.

A more serious consideration is that drugs to calm children can be the precursor of stronger medication which eventually leads to the introduction of street drugs and the child's addiction. This leads to the eventual destruction of the adolescent and the cataclysmic problems of the sorrowful parents. Many drug problems later in life can be traced back to this type prescription drug.

ALTERNATIVE NATURAL REMEDIES

Eliminate foods containing natural salicylates as listed above.

Avoid taking aspirin which is a salicylate.

Diet control is of the utmost importance. Eliminate all junk food, fast food, cookies, cake, ice cream, sodas and candy. Since a child cannot be watched 24 hours a day, this is often an unrealistic approach to the problem. It must be initiated slowly, since taking away all a child's "goodies" at once could have a negative effect. The child would then rebel and consume some forbidden foods secretly.

If a child is on medication, tests should be performed to see if there is an allergy to any of the ingredients.

All sugars and products containing sugars should be removed from the diet of a hyperactive child. This includes white sugar, honey, molasses, maple syrup, fructose, dextrose, corn syrup, lactose (from milk), mannitol, sorbitol (candy sweeteners), xylitol (chewing gum sweetener) and synthetic sweeteners such as saccharine and Nutra Sweet. Some studies have shown that Nutra Sweet may increase hyperactivity in certain people, who may be allergic to the phenylalanine in it.

Try to pack lunch rather than allowing the child to buy it in the school cafeteria where the majority of foods are not nutritious, but are highly sweetened and absolutely worthless to the health aspects of a growing child. Cooperation of the child is essential.

Children are bombarded by the media, with ads stressing the positive aspects of sugary and junk foods. This is not an easy problem to solve. Parents of these children should consider forming a support group to work on the authorities for a change in the advertising system.

A deficiency in nutrients should be addressed. A children's multi-vitamin/mineral combination usually makes up for the lack of nutrients. The best diet is one consisting of natural type foods such as whole grains instead of white flour products, brown rice instead of white rice, green leafy vegetables, salads, and fruits without salycilates. Also include starchy vegetables grown underground, fish, organic chicken and turkey and cultured or fermented organic dairy products such as yogurt, sour cream, cottage cheese and other cheeses. Do not include milk because many children are highly allergic to it, and the lactose (milk sugar) causes hyperactivity. When dairy products are cultured and fermented, the sugar content is changed.

Supplements

Vitamin C, 1000 mg. to 3000 mg. daily.

Pantothene, 200 mg. three times daily.

Niacin, 500 mg. twice daily (causes some flushing).

These supplements help activate the immune system to fight the deleterious effects of processed foods and chemicals.

Herbs

Borage oil, 1 capsule containing 240 mg. of G.L.A. twice daily, lowers allergic reactions.

Hops acts as a calmative and lowers hyperexcitability to the nervous system, alleviates nervous tension and promotes restful sleep. It acts as a sedative in place of medicine.

Skullcap helps control nervous disorders and relaxes the brain.

Valerian root acts as a tranquilizer.

Passion flower soothes nerves and relaxes the body.

Amino Acids

L-Taurine, 500 mg. twice daily on empty stomach, is a calming neurotransmitter.

GABA, 500 mg. twice daily on empty stomach, has an anti-anxiety effect.

Adjunctive Modalities

Parents must take control of the child rather than allowing the child to control them. They must stop trying to please the child at every turn because eventually this causes the child to lose respect and love for the parents, leading to a maladjusted personality as the child matures. Just as juvenile diabetics must follow a special diet, hyperactive children must also watch what they eat.

HYPOGLYCEMIA (LOW BLOOD SUGAR)

DEFINITION

An abnormally low level of blood sugar causing the body and brain's energy levels to become incapacitated. This may lead to extreme fatigue and possibly coma and death. An insensitivity to one's own insulin causes it to overproduce to the degree that the body calls for more glucose, causing sugar cravings. High insulin levels remove too much sugar from the blood, resulting in abnormally low blood sugar levels.

CAUSES

Overconsumption of sugary type foods.

Insensitivity and overproduction of insulin from the pancreas, due to less functional islet cells.

Raising blood sugar too quickly, causing its rapid lowering (crashing).

Diabetics on insulin must regulate the dosage and adjust it so too much is not taken, lowering blood sugar to the point of coma.

CONVENTIONAL TREATMENT

This condition is not recognized as a disease by the orthodoxy.

PROBLEMS ASSOCIATED WITH CONVENTIONAL TREATMENT

Diagnostic procedures for this condition are usually not done by the orthodoxy, but they are definitely recommended for a true diagnosis of this disease. A three hour glucose tolerance test is not sufficient. A six hour test must be done.

This is performed by having the patient drink two ounces of a pure sugar solution and drawing blood samples in 30 minutes and then every hour for six hours. A graph is plotted to determine high and low sugar levels. This graph must be interpreted by someone who has the ability to understand differences in the time elements of these highs and lows.

A reading below 50 indicates hypoglycemia. A reading above 190 at the beginning of the test could be a sign of a pre-diabetic condition. A faint or shaky condition of the patient during the test must also be taken into consideration as it would indicate low blood sugar.

Hypoglycemia can be a precursor to diabetes. Both conditions are caused by malfunctioning islet cells of the pancreas.

ALTERNATIVE NATURAL REMEDIES

Diet

A high protein, low carbohydrate diet must be followed. The reason is that more insulin is needed to digest carbohydrates than proteins. Eat foods high in protein (one gram for every two pounds of body weight), low in processed carbohydrates. and high in fiber. High fiber foods form a gel in the intestinal tract that may hold or trap sugar for a period of time so it will be more slowly absorbed into the intestines. Complex carbohydrates are foods grown in the field, such as fruits, greens, grains, starchy vegetables, nuts and seeds. These all convert to glucose which must be carried into the cell with insulin to produce cellular energy. With fewer carbohydrates ingested, less insulin will be needed, thereby lowering the hypoglycemic reaction.

Foods aiding normal insulin production are:

Cucumbers, which contain a hormone needed by cells of the pancreas to produce insulin.

Onions and garlic, which contain natural beneficial hormones.

Jerusalem artichokes, which stimulate insulin production.

String bean juice or string bean pod tea, which help keep glucose under control.

Proteins and fats from fish, fowl, meat and dairy products are converted into energy through a different chemical pathway that uses much less insulin. Thus the pancreas is not weakened by overproducing insensitive insulin. Eat more fish, organic white meat chicken and turkey without skin, veal, lamb, lean pork, non-fat cottage and Swiss cheese, plain yogurt, butter, soft cooked or poached eggs and lean organic beef. Avocados, olives, macademia nuts, salads and green leafy type vegetables are allowed.

Many patients, especially those with poor digestion, do better eating small meals three hours apart. Cooked grains take twice as long as raw grains to digest.

Supplements

Chromium picolinate, 200 mcg. three times daily, enhances glucose and insulin's ability to enter the cell and produce energy (ATP) in the cell.

Zinc picolinate, 30 mg. twice daily, is a component of insulin and helps enhance its sensitivity to glucose.

Manganese, 50 mg. twice daily. A deficiency in this mineral can affect glucose tolerance.

Magnesium citrate, 400 mg. three times daily, is a component of insulin.

Vitamin C, 500 mg. four times daily, helps normalize sugar metabolism.

B complex, 50 mg. twice daily, increases tolerance to sugars and carbohydrates.

Pantothene, (B6), 300 mg. three times daily, strengthens exhausted adrenal glands, a condition common among hypoglycemics.

Vitamin E, 200 I.U., building up to 800 I.U. slowly, aids glycogen storage in the liver and muscle tissues.

Digestive multiple enzymes (Pancreatin), 1 or 2 with each meal, insures proper breakdown of food.

Herbs

Licorice supplies quick energy.

Safflower aids the pancreas in its manufacture of natural insulin.

Amino Acids

L-Taurine, 500 mg. four times daily on an empty stomach, potentiates action of insulin and moderates blood sugar levels.

L-Tryptophan, 500 mg. three times daily (from pure sources), reduces carbohydrate cravings.

L-Alanine, per label, is a major energy precursor.

L-Arginine, 1000 mg. three times daily, moderates glucose tolerance.

L-Glutathione, 100 mg. three times daily on empty stomach, is a glucose tolerance factor.

L-Glutamine, 500 mg. four times daily on empty stomach, reduces cravings for sugar.

L-Lysine, 500 mg. twice daily on empty stomach, promotes insulin production.

Adjunctive Modalities

Freeze-dried glandular pancreas enhances insulin production. It is not the insulin that causes the problem. It is the quality, and if it is too insensitive, the pancreas overproduces it.

IMPOTENCE

DEFINITION

The inability for a male to achieve or maintain an erection or have a normal ejaculation. (Erection is not necessary for orgasm or ejaculation.)

CAUSES

Medications used to treat high blood pressure.

Medications used to treat ulcers.

Antihistamines.

Antidepressants.

Tranquilizers decrease sex drive and cause nerve blockage.

Chemotherapy for cancer which leads to generalized weakness.

Estrogen used in treatment of prostate cancer.

Narcotics decrease libido.

Alcoholism.

Organic nervous conditions.

Psychological nervous conditions.

Lowered pineal gland and hypocampus function.

Low blood sugar.

Overconsumption of caffeine.

Scar tissue from previous surgery in gonadal area.

Hypothyroidism.

Hypogonadism.

Decreased hormonal levels.

Smoking can lower testosterone levels and cause accumulation of large amounts of carbon dioxide which decreases the amount of oxygen delivered to the cells. An insufficient amount of oxygen in the cells causes them to become dysfunctional. Smoking also constricts small arteries in the gonadal area causing a decreased blood supply.

Steroids used to improve muscle function and form in athletes and weight lifters eventually cause the testicles to shrink.

Eating food containing DES (Diethylstilbestrol), the growth hormone fed to animals and poultry, causes destruction of virility in men.

This is the same hormone that causes vaginal cancer in the daughters of women who took the drug during pregnancy to prevent miscarriages.

Heating of the genitals by saunas or hot tubs or wearing tight pants slows the production of male hormones.

CONVENTIONAL TREATMENT

Hormonal therapy.

Psychotherapy.

Surgery—Implantation of penile prosthesis, either rigid or semi-flexible or inflatable devices.

PROBLEMS ASSOCIATED WITH CONVENTIONAL TREATMENT

Side effects of hormonal therapy can cause other problems in your system that may be even worse than the original situation.

Surgery is not always successful and leaves scar tissue which causes problems later in life.

ALTERNATIVE NATURAL REMEDIES

Diet

Eating oysters and clams were an old folk remedy for curing impotence. Although I do not recommend eating shellfish due to their toxic content, there is some merit to this remedy. Oysters and clams are rich in zinc, an important mineral for prostate gland function, normal sperm count and sexual libido. Other good sources of zinc are wheat germ and organ meats.

Supplements

High potency multi-vitamin/mineral combination once daily.

Zinc picolinate, 30 mg. twice daily.

Vitamin E, 400 I.U. once daily.

Vitamin C, 500 mg. four times daily.

Beta carotene A, 25,000 I.U. once daily.

Gerovital, an anti-aging supplement from Roumania. Take according to directions on label.

Herbs

Licorice is a stimulant.

Damiana increases sperm count.

Sarsaparilla stimulates circulation.

Capsicum stimulates other herbs to go to the location where they are needed.

Siberian ginseng contains testosterone to help correct impotence.

Saw palmetto nourishes the reproductive glands.

Ginko biloba helps with the circulation of blood to the testical area.

Amino Acids

L-Arginine, 1000 mg. three times daily on empty stomach, is good for formation and activity of sperm. A high sperm count often helps activate libido.

L-Histadine, 500 mg. twice daily on empty stomach, is an excellent carrier for zinc.

Adjunctive Therapy

Men who fear not being able to perform to the expectations of their partner are with the wrong person, and should definitely make a change. Unless you are with someone who makes you feel comfortable and at ease, you will have problems.

INSOMNIA

DEFINITION

Insomnia is the inability to fall asleep within a normal amount of time, which is about five to ten minutes. It is also the inability to stay asleep without awakening two to three hours after going to sleep. Individual amounts of sleep vary from person to person, depending on basic energy needs. The body requires less sleep as it grows older than it did while in a growing state.

While sleeping, the brain is the part of the body that is at rest and, without enough sleep, people become irritable and anxious. The rest of the body does not require sleep. Studies have shown certain people do not require any sleep at all because their systems have the ability to repair brain damage without sleep.

CAUSES

Medical problems such as diabetes, headaches, migraine headaches, asthma, ulcers, and under or overactive thyroid (hypothyroidism, or hyperthyroidism).

Environmental problems such as noise, poor mattress, temperature changes, dryness from hot air heat (it can cause relative humidity to go down to 15 percent, which is lower than the humidity in Death Valley), position of bed according to polar direction, north/south compared to east/west.

Dietary considerations such as low blood sugar, too much caffeine or alcoholic beverages, spicy foods, allergy causing foods and MSG. Improper digestion which causes deficiencies in vitamins, minerals, amino acids and enzymes needed for a healthy body. Too much salt which stimulates the adrenal glands and can cause the overproduction of adrenalin.

Psychological problems such as not being able to relax, worrying, anxiety and tension brought on by the demands of everyday living.

Sleep apnea and snoring.

Respiratory disorders such as asthma, emphysema and bronchitis.

Nightmares and sleepwalking.

Low serotonin levels in the brain.

CONVENTIONAL TREATMENT

Sleep inducing medications.

Tranquilizers.

Psychotherapy.

Behavior modification.

Workup at sleep disorder center.

PROBLEMS ASSOCIATED WITH CONVENTIONAL TREATMENT

Medications become so addictive that you have problems falling asleep naturally. Medications can also cause dizziness, swelling of eyelids, slow heartbeat, unusual excitement, sore throat and fever.

ALTERNATIVE NATURAL REMEDIES

Diet

A well-balanced diet will enhance overall health and allow for normal sleeping. Sleep-inducing foods are dairy products, eggs, salmon, turkey, chicken and lamb which are high in tryptophan and tyrosine.

Avoid alcohol, sugar and foods with a high sugar content before bedtime as they cause the blood sugar to plummet, leading to improper sleep patterns.

Do not eat spicy foods or beans, which can lead to indigestion, burping, heartburn and flatulence, and disturb normal sleep patterns.

The body should be in an alkaline state when sleeping at night. An acid state generally prevails during waking hours. To make the body more alkaline, take one teaspoon of powdered or liquid green in the form of green magma, wheat grass or barley grass in eight ounces of water an hour before retiring. If you prefer, you can drink a glass of green vegetable juice.

Supplements

Vitamin B complex deficiencies should be addressed since they act as a calming agent in the body.

Vitamin C and Vitamin B6 are necessary to convert tryptophan to serotonin, the neurotransmitter that promotes normal sleep.

The following supplements all calm nerves and promote sleep.

Vitamin C, 500 mg. four times daily.

Vitamin B6, 100 mg. three times daily.

Magnesium citrate, 500 mg. three times daily.

Potassium citrate, 99 mg. five times daily.

Calcium citrate, 500 mg. twice daily.

Chronoset (melatonin, a neurotransmitter), 2 mg. before retiring normalizes circadian rhythms.

Herbs

Valerian root acts as a tranquilizer.

Skullcap relaxes the mind.

Hops reduces restlessness and aids in producing sleep.

Blue vervian is a natural tranquilizer.

Camomile is good for the nerves.

Lady Slipper is a tonic for an exhausted nervous system and has a calming effect on the body and mind.

Passion flower weans you from synthetic tranquilizers and sleeping pills, and it is quieting and soothing to the nervous system.

Amino Acids

GABA reduces sleeplessness.

Tryptophan (from pure sources) is a precursor of serotonin, a calming neurotransmitter. (Or snack on pumpkin seeds in the evening. Eight ounces supply 1250 mg. of tryptophan.)

Adjunctive Methods

Aligning the body in the proper polar direction helps many people get a better night's sleep. North/south vs. east/west can have a de-stimulating effect on the body's electrical energy. Try reversing sleeping position 90 degrees or switch the head and foot of the bed.

Take a leisurely walk one hour before bedtime.

Warm baths are relaxing.

Light massages soothe the body.

A 10 to 15 minute meditation period before bedtime does wonders in bringing about a feeling of restfulness at the day's end.

Try changing your philosophy to just getting through one day at a time. The future has a way of taking care of itself if you take care of yourself.

Calming new age type music and relaxation tapes help induce sleep. Be sure you have the type of tape recorder that shuts off quietly when the tape is done.

Sexual activity with the right person can relieve tensions and promote sleep.

Avoid cured meats, potatoes, tomatoes, eggplant, sauerkraut and spinach because they contain tyramine which increases the release of a brain chemical stimulant.

Avoid coffee, tea and chocolate after noon.

KIDNEY STONES

DEFINITION

An abnormal accumulation of mineral salts that are formulated in the kidneys. There are three types of kidney stones:

Stones formed from calcium oxalic acid are the most prevalent. Oxalic acids are derived from rhubarb, tea, dairy products, nuts and dark green leafy vegetables such as spinach, chard and kale.

Stones formed from uric acid.

Stones formed from cystine, the result of consuming too much protein.

Symptoms are severe pain in the lower back, radiating to the bladder area in the lower front part of the abdomen. Pain is excruciating when the stone is exiting from the kidney into the ureter. It then tries to work its way down the ureter to the bladder and out of the body. Some types of kidney stones (staghorn) grow to such a large size that they are unable to exit the kidney. These stones will eventually block the filtration mechanism in the kidney and will have to be removed surgically.

The male ureter has a bend near its center that can trap a stone, causing urine to back up into the kidney causing severe pain. The intensity of pain from kidney stones is compared to that of the final stages of labor. Many men lose consciousness from the pain.

Stones can take from 15 minutes to six weeks to pass from one end of the urinary tract to the other. They can lead to bladder and kidney infections. Some stones are of miniscule size (gravel or sand) and pass through the urinary tract painlessly.

CAUSES

A deficiency in magnesium causes urine to have a high alkaline content which results in the formation of stones. Magnesium balances calcium in the system. If calcium is not balanced, it can proliferate, store in the kidneys and form stones.

A deficiency in Vitamin B6 raises oxalic acid and increases alkalinity.

Diets too low in protein produce albumin which prevents calcium from being excreted properly and it accumulates in the kidneys.

Vitamin D helps metabolize calcium. Too little causes a decrease in calcium absorption, resulting in the accumulation of calcium deposits in the kidneys. Conversely, too much Vitamin D overmetabolizes calcium, causing it to collect in the kidneys. Some women are prescribed megadoses of Vitamin D for osteoporosis. They must be monitored carefully.

Cystine buildup due to a hereditary disease can form large stones in the kidneys.

An imbalance in the ratio between calcium and phosphorus (which should be 1 part phosphorus to 2.5 parts calcium) will cause an alkaline condition in the body favorable for stone formation. People who take large amounts of antacids are getting too much calcium carbonate into their bodies. Calcium carbonate is an inorganic substance that is difficult to absorb, especially with aging, as fewer digestive acids and enzymes are formed in the stomach and intestinal tract.

An overactive parathyroid gland raises calcium in the bloodstream.

Too much calcium from food, particularly dairy products, sardines with bones, and dark green leafy vegetables such as spinach, chard, kale and turnip greens.

CONVENTIONAL TREATMENT

Removal of stones by surgery.

Removal of stones through a lighted tube inserted into the urethra.

Lithotripsy, a relatively new method in which stones are bombarded with ultrasonic radiation to make them smaller and easier to pass.

Medication to dissolve stones.

PROBLEMS ASSOCIATED WITH CONVENTIONAL TREATMENT.

The cause is not removed, and stones continue to form. With aging, stones can cause irreparable damage to tissues. Side effects of medication can destroy kidney tissues to the point where it cannot repair itself. Medication depresses the immune system to the degree of causing autoimmune disease. Total loss of kidney function can result in uremic poisoning and death.

ALTERNATIVE NATURAL REMEDIES

Diet

Although too much protein leads to excessive amounts of calcium in the kidneys, moderate amounts are necessary to produce sufficient albumin, which keeps calcium in solution. The average adult should consume 55 grams of pure protein daily. Protein varies according to the type of food ingested. Those who do not eat animal type foods should be aware of food combinations that add up to complete proteins which are necessary to sustain life. Tape a food composition chart (available in health food stores) on your refrigerator door.

Do not drink too much milk since it is fortified with Vitamin D, which causes a higher absorption of calcium into the system, and it is a synthetic form of Vitamin D which is inorganic to the body. It is also too high in phosphorus which slows the breakdown of calcium.

Avoid foods with a high oxalic acid content such as dark green leafy vegetables, dairy products, chocolate, rhubarb, tea, nuts and seeds. Foods in the cabbage family and beets produce oxalic acid.

The best vegetables for the kidneys are parsley, cucumber, celery, horseradish, watercress, asparagus and garlic. They help the body rid itself of inorganic matter by increasing liver activity.

Bananas and papaya have a healing effect on the kidneys.

Watermelon and watermelon juice are excellent for flushing the kidneys.

Cranberry juice has an antiseptic effect.

Pears help relieve inflammatory conditions such as nephritis.

Drink at least two quarts of distilled water daily. You know you are drinking enough water if at least once a day your urine is clear, not yellow. Then the kidneys have been properly flushed.

Supplements

Vitamin B6, 100 mg. three times daily, acts as a diuretic.

Magnesium citrate, 400 mg. twice daily and Vitamin B2, 100 mg. twice daily, are needed to insure proper absorption of B6.

Vitamin A, fish liver, 25,000 I.U. and Beta carotene, 25,000 I.U., are needed to fend off accumulation of kidney stones.

Phosphorus, per label, raises body acidity and dissolves blood calcium so it does not store in your kidneys.

Vitamin C, 1000 mg. four times daily, helps keep urine in an acid state.

Lecithin, 1200 mg. six times daily, helps purify the kidneys.

Vitamin E, 400 I.U., helps clear up kidney problems.

Zinc picolinate, 30 mg. twice daily, has a positive effect on alkaline acid balance.

Multi-vitamin/mineral combination, once daily.

Herbs

Marshmallow helps remove mucous from kidneys and is soothing to the urinary tract. Mucous in organs causes blockage.

Ginger aids in kidney cleansing.

Parsley tones up the urinary system.

Uva ursi acts as a solvent to urinic calculi deposits.

Comfrey aids in balancing calcium and phosphorus.

Golden seal aids in eliminating toxins from the kidneys. Do not use this herb if there are blood sugar problems. Use dandelion root instead.

Corn silk tea is a natural diuretic.

Shepherd's purse is a natural diuretic.

Dyer's root (madder) may dissolve kidney stones.

Amino Acid

L-Glutathione, 100 mg. three times daily on an empty stomach, increases renal clearance of uric acid.

LEG CRAMPS
(INTERMITTENT CLAUDICATION)

DEFINITION

The slowing of blood circulation to the lower extremities causing pain.

CAUSES

Arteriosclerosis, hardening of the arteries.

Atherosclerosis, narrowing of the arteries from interior blockage.

Heart disease. Weakened condition of the heart slows the pumping action needed for blood to reach the lower extremities.

Thickened blood.

Blood containing too much fat or cholesterol.

Heredity factors.

Low estrogen levels in women.

Smoking, which contracts arteries and capillaries.

High blood pressure.

Little or no exercise.

Overweight.

Sugar imbalance, either diabetes or hypoglycemia.

Undue stress.

CONVENTIONAL TREATMENT

Diagnostic procedures to determine state of blood flow. One type is angiography, where a catheter is inserted into an artery of the lower extremity. Doppler testing is a method using sound waves.

Bypass surgery of arteries in the lower extremities.

Removal of blockage in arteries.

Sympathectomy, the severing of nerves to the arteries to help improve circulation.

Medications to dilate blood vessels.

Small amounts, about one ounce of whiskey or brandy has a dilating effect on blood vessels.

Weight loss.

Low fat diet.

Exercise to improve circulation. At least one hour walking daily, jogging, swimming, cycling, walking in waist high water.

PROBLEMS ASSOCIATED WITH CONVENTIONAL TREATMENT

A diagnostic angiogram is a surgical procedure entailing a hospital stay, side effects of anesthesia and stress.

Bypass surgery addresses only the immediate symptom without reversing the problem. If arterial destruction and disruption is not addressed, it will proliferate and the original condition can return.

Sympathectomy has side effects, including possible loss of feeling and sensation from severing nerves.

Medication to dilate blood vessels in the legs also dilates vessels in the entire body, causing overactivity of the blood supply in some of the wrong areas.

ALTERNATIVE NATURAL REMEDIES

Diet

To lower the fat content of blood, eliminate all foods with a high fat content including animal fats, dairy fats, poultry skin, fatty fish such as bluefish, salmon, lobster and shrimp.

Avoid consuming sugar which eventually turns to fat. Besides white sugar, refrain from eating foods that convert into glucose in the body such as sweet fruits, including grapes, bananas, citrus, watermelon, cantaloupe and honeydew. Do not eat cookies, cake, candy, ice cream, junk food, processed food or chocolate. Fruit juices also have a high sugar content.

Season foods with cayenne red pepper, horseradish, garlic and ginger. They act as vasodilators and aid circulation.

Supplements

Vitamin E helps thin the blood. Start taking 200 I.U. daily for one week. Each week add 200 I.U. until a dose of 1200 I.U. is reached. Building up the amount in this fashion will prevent a rise in blood pressure.

Niacin, 100 mg. three times daily. Gradually increase dose over a six week period until taking 1000 mg. daily. This acts as a vasodilator and blood thinner.

Fish oil (Omega 3), 1000 mg. six times daily, thins blood and prevents platelets from adhering to each other.

Bromelain, 500 mg. twice daily, acts as an anti-inflammatory.

Pantothene, 300 mg. three times daily, helps the body produce its own anti-inflammatory agents such as cortisol.

Calcium citrate, 800 mg. and magnesium citrate, 1200 mg., assist in the contraction and expansion of muscles surrounding the arteries.

Good quality multi-vitamin/mineral combination once daily.

Herbs

Comfrey helps regulate calcium phosphorus balance, promotes strong bones and healthy arteries.

Cramp bark helps potassium, calcium, magnesium balance which alleviates muscle cramping.

Capsicum is a vasodilator.

Cloves increase circulation of blood.

Amino Acids

L-Histadine, per directions on label, is a powerful vasodilator.

Adjunctive Methods

Castor oil packs. Soak a piece of white flannel in warm castor oil, wring it out and place over the painful area. Cover with plastic and apply a heating pad. Do this twice a day for one hour each sitting.

Light massage therapy.

Acupuncture.

MENOPAUSE

DEFINITION

The cessation of menstruation and ovulation accompanied by a lowering in the production of female hormones. The time period from the beginning of menstruation until menopause is usually 35 years. Nowadays, in the United States, the average female starts menstruating between the ages of 11 and 13. In the mid-nineteenth century, the average age was 17 due to a lower sugar and fat intake in the diet, which kept estrogen levels low.

Estrogen is a fat soluble hormone that resides in fatty tissue. A high body fat content causes more production and storage of estrogen, leading to an earlier onset of menstruation. High fat content in the body may be a precipitating factor in setting the stage for a precancerous tumor.

Menstrual changes are one of the early symptoms of menopause. The flow can be lighter, heavier, occur more or less frequently, or stop abruptly. Menopausal symptoms usually last about five years. Some, but not all women suffer from hot flashes, night sweats, vaginal and vulvar dryness.

Although many women complain of irritability, depression and difficulty sleeping during the menopausal years, there is no clinical evidence for these complaints. More than likely these symptoms are caused by sleep deprivation due to hot flashes.

Decreased estrogen production may lead to osteoporosis, a condition of increased bone porosity. The reason estrogen protects against bone loss is that it helps to metabolize copper, which is necessary to manufacture bone. Women actually do become shorter due to compression of the spinal column. When the upper spine is affected, women acquire "dowager's hump." Spontaneous fractures may occur.

Prior to menopause, the rate of heart attacks is less for women than for men, because estrogen has some protective factor. Without estrogen, women have a greater risk of heart attacks.

CAUSES

Normal aging process.

A deficiency in hormones from the pituitary gland could initiate an early menopause.

Disturbances in calcium metabolism (calcium becomes insoluble and is not absorbed into the system).

CONVENTIONAL TREATMENT

Hormone replacement therapy with estrogen and progesterone.

PROBLEMS ASSOCIATED WITH CONVENTIONAL TREATMENT

Cancer of the endometrium.

Increased risk of breast cancer.

Gallbladder disease.

High blood pressure.

Synthetic estrogen is fifteen times as strong as your body's estrogen. You are told hormone replacement therapy is safe, yet doctors insist that you be carefully monitored. Women who cannot avoid taking estrogen and have had hepatitis or other liver problems, should use the estrogen patch. This delivery system bypasses the liver. A side effect may be an allergic reaction to the skin.

ALTERNATIVE NATURAL REMEDIES

Diet

Maintain normal weight. Women should weigh 100 pounds for the first five feet and five pounds more for every inch over five feet. For example a woman who is five feet four inches tall should weigh 120 pounds. Weight can vary a few pounds according to body size, which can be determined by taking the middle finger and thumb of one hand and encircling the opposite wrist. If the fingers touch, bone size is medium. If they overlap, bone size is small, and if there is a space, bone size is large.

The best way to lose weight is to go on a high protein, low carbohydrate diet. Avoid fruit, juices, breads, pastas, white flour, starchy vegetables such as potatoes, beets, yams, carrots, rice and corn. Eliminate all sugars, cookies, candy, cake, ice cream, soda, chocolate and pastries. Eliminate cheese steaks, pizza, fast foods, pretzels or crackers. Once normal weight is attained, small amounts of these foods may be consumed on a staggered basis. For more information on weight loss, consult the chapter entitled OBESITY.

Those who are too thin may enter menopause at an earlier age because of lessened estrogen production. Women often get too thin from undereating, overexercising or psychological factors such as having perfectionist type personalities. Anorexics and bulemics also have decreased hormone production.

The underweight, overly-thin woman should try to bring her weight up to normal by increasing her intake of complex carbohydrate foods such as fruits, whole grains, nuts, seeds, starchy vegetables and salads.

The following foods have a high folic acid content which increases natural estrogen production: legumes, endive, oats, sunflower seeds, liver, brewer's yeast, wheat germ and alfalfa.

Foods containing large amounts of estrogen are cow's milk, eggs, meat from animals raised on hormones, carrots, yams and pomegranate seeds.

Wild Mexican yams produce progesterone.

Foods for thyroid gland stimulation are potatoes, apples, mushrooms and sesame seeds. Reduced thyroid function leads to overweight. A normally functioning or slightly overactive thyroid helps burn unwanted fat.

Supplements

Folic acid, 10 mg. to 60 mg. produces estrogen in the body. However the highest amount available without a prescription is 400 to 800 mcg. One thousand micrograms are equal to one milligram. Since high amounts of folic acid in the body can mask symptoms of pernicious anemia, the FDA does not allow the health food industry to manufacture a higher strength capsule or tablet. Only a holistic physician will prescribe the high amounts of folic acid and monitor the patient.

PABA, 500 mg. twice daily, increases estrogen.

Boron, 3 mg. three times daily, protects against bone loss.

Good quality multi-vitamin/mineral supplement such as VM75 once daily.

Vitamin B6, 100 mg. three times daily, enhances the effect of existing estrogen.

Pantothene, 300 mg. three times daily, acts as a precursor to the production of estrogen from the adrenal glands.

Note: Even though your ovaries have stopped producing estrogen, when your adrenal glands are stimulated to a high enough degree they can produce small amounts of estrogen.

Before menopause, you had thinner blood because you became mildly anemic during menstruation. The thinner blood protected you from heart attacks. Therefore it is essential that you take the following blood thinning supplements:

Omega 3 fish oil, 6 capsules daily.

Garlic, 4 capsules daily.

Niacin, 200 mg. twice daily. (Flushing may occur.)

Vitamin C, 1000 mg. three times daily.

Vitamin E, start with 200 I.U. and work up to 1200 to 1600 I.U. over a two-month period.

The above supplements are organic to the body which means they are utilized in a natural state. There is a natural feedback system within the body. When the body manufactures its own chemicals and decides enough has been made, it stops the output, preventing overproduction and avoiding side effects. Inorganic materials such as Premarin (estrogen) and Provera (progesterone) are not affected by the body's feedback system, leading to too large a degree of buildup of these materials. This leads to deleterious and long lasting side effects such as blood clots, diabetes, liver problems and depression.

Herbs

Anise produces estrogen.

Dong Quai relieves hot flashes.

Mexican wild yam helps produce progesterone.

Licorice, parsley, comfrey and yarrow help maintain proper blood viscosity.

Change of Life Formula, per label. This is an excellent product consisting of:

Black cohash, which contains natural estrogen and helps alleviate hot flashes.

Sarsaparilla, which contains progesterone.

Siberian ginseng, which corrects hormonal imbalance.

Licorice root, which stimulates the adrenal glands.

False unicorn, which stimulates the reproductive organs.

Squaw vine, which helps kidney function.

Adjunctive Methods

Vitamin E oil, applied topically for vaginal dryness.

Vitamin A, D, E cream, for vaginal dryness.

Note: An interesting fact is that nicotine promotes estrogen buildup. However this is not to recommend that menopausal women take up smoking since the risks outweigh the benefits.

MULTIPLE SCLEROSIS

DEFINITION

The deterioration of the myelin sheath, the insulation that covers nerves and neurons, which are the electrical message sending units of the central nervous system. MS stands for multiple scarring, a process which eventually stops nerve impulses. Early symptoms are tremors, bladder and bowel disturbances, paralysis, an unsteady gait, speech slurring and other sensory impairments.

This disease is more likely to occur among populations in the temperate zones rather than in the tropics or polar areas. It usually starts during the teens or early twenties and in rare cases can occur after age forty.

CAUSES

An autoimmune disorder. Under normal circumstances, the patient's immune system perceives a particular virus, attacks it, defeats it and at the proper time withdraws its defenders. When the immune system malfunctions, the system continues to attack, destroying not only the virus, but also in this case, the myelin sheath.

Lack of Vitamin D which is needed for repair of the demyelinated sheath. Sunlight on the skin combines with cholesterol to produce Vitamin D. More cases are diagnosed in the winter since less sunlight is available.

Multiple sclerosis patients have eight times the amount of mercury in their spinal fluid. Mercury is a demyelinating substance, it worsens multiple sclerosis. Most mercury stored in your body is derived from amalgam fillings in the teeth. Fifty two percent of these fillings consist of mercury. These fillings must be removed in order to help you go into remission. This must be performed by an experienced dentist well versed in the procedure. Otherwise the problem will be exacerbated. For further information on this subject, contact Dr. Hal Huggins at 1-800-331-2303.

Environmental sensitivities such as molds, fungi, pollens, dust and chemicals.

Heavy metal toxicity such as lead, aluminum, cadmium and arsenic.

Platinum from the catalytic convertor in automobiles.

More cases are diagnosed in heavily industrialized areas.

Food allergies.

Lack of lecithin.

Low copper, iodine, manganese and sulfur.

Carbon monoxide pollution.

High fat diet impairs conversion of linoleic acid to prostaglandin (E1), the anti-inflammatory prostaglandin.

If a pregnant woman is deficient in linoleic acid, she can increase the child's susceptibility to the demyelinating factor which can eventually cause the disease.

Oxidation of saturated oils, particularly palm and coconut, into free radicals which attack the myelin sheath.

The number of cases of multiple sclerosis has tripled in the past 20 years due to fluoridated water, which depresses the immune system. Fluorine is a drug that was incorporated into the water supply without our consent.

CONVENTIONAL TREATMENT

High tech diagnostic procedures such as M.R.I.

Steroids.

PROBLEMS ASSOCIATED WITH CONVENTIONAL TREATMENT

Side effects of steroids are:

Depletion of calcium which is needed to help control M.S.

Water retention.

Electrolyte imbalance causing loss of minerals, specifically calcium, magnesium and potassium, which are needed for repair of the myelin cells. These cells regulate fluid excretion which helps normalize blood pressure.

Stomach ulcers.

Psychosis.

ALTERNATIVE NATURAL REMEDIES

Diet

Eat natural foods only. Avoid all processed, preserved, or denatured food, sugar and junk food.

The lactose in milk increases absorption and retention of lead. Skim milk contains the most lactose. Cream or 4 percent milk has less.

Eliminate alcohol and stop smoking, since both destroy B vitamins and worsen symptoms.

Vegetables, fruits, whole grains, starches fish, chicken, and eggs must all be organic.

Use only polyunsaturated oils such as safflower or canola.

Whey, the liquid portion of soured or curdled milk, contains Vitamin B13 (orotic acid) which has been shown to aid in the treatment of M.S.

Supplements

Omega 3 fatty acids (fish oils), 1000 mg. six times daily.

Omega 6 fatty acids, Evening primrose oil, 2 capsules three times daily, or Borage oil, 1 capsule three times daily.

Vitamin E, 200 I.U. to start, and gradually build up to 1800 I.U. over a three month period.

Phosphatidyl choline (from lecithin), take double the amount suggested on the label. Lecithin has been found lacking in the brain of multiple sclerosis patients.

Inositol, 500 mg., three times daily. People with M.S. are usually deficient in this. It also has a calming effect on the central nervous system.

Cod liver oil, 1 tsp. twice daily.

Copper, 2 to 4 mg. daily.

B complex, 100 mg., one daily.

Vitamin B6, 100 mg. three times daily.

Vitamin B1, 100 mg. three times daily, as an anti-inflammatory.

Magnesium citrate, 400 mg. three times daily, aids in eliminating spasms, twitching and poor bladder control.

Vitamin B12, 500 mcg. three times daily, increases stability in standing and walking.

Octacosanol, 5 mg. daily, improves muscle control.

Note: High doses of Vitamin C are not prescribed for M.S. patients because it increases carbon dioxide in the blood. People with M.S. have problems with oxygen transfer in the lungs because of membrane disease.

Adenosine #5, monophosphate (must be prescribed by holistic physician.)

Calcium EAP (by Dr. Hans Neiper of Germany. To order call 1-800-53-LOGIC). This should be administered intravenously by a holistic physician. It is one of the best known supplements for fighting the effects of autoimmune diseases.

Amino Acids

N-Acetyl Cysteine, 1200 mg. every other day, chelates mucous, heavy metals and toxins from the body.

L-Isoleucine and leucine, per label, are major sources of energy for muscles and reduce stress to the central nervous system.

L-Lysine, 500 mg. twice daily on empty stomach, reduces the inflammatory response of antibodies (for autoimmune response).

D-Phenylalanine, 500 mg. twice daily on empty stomach, for bladder control.

Adjunctive Methods

Hyperbaric oxygen. This is a system of utilizing 100 percent oxygen. The patient sits in a tent-like enclosure for three hours while oxygen from a tank is pumped in. This enhances oxygen metabolism. These units are available to rent. For further information, call the M.S. Society in your area.

Massage and swimming help activate the lymphatic system. This in turn helps eliminate the toxins that cause slowdown of muscle control which is already impaired in your body.

OBESITY

DEFINITION

Obesity is the state of having an excessive amount of fat on the body. Anyone whose weight is twenty percent more than it should be is considered obese. One way to determine ideal weight is to allow 100 pounds for the first five feet of height and add five pounds for each inch over five feet. Since muscle weighs more than fat, athletic types may weigh more.

To ascertain frame size, take the thumb and middle finger of the right hand and encircle the left wrist. If they overlap, you are small boned. If they meet, you are medium boned. If there is a space between the thumb and finger, you are large boned. You may add five to ten pounds to your ideal weight if you are large boned. Subtract five to ten pounds if you are small boned.

CAUSES

Inability to metabolize food at a normal rate due to diseases such as diabetes, hypothyroidism or low blood sugar.

Lack of exercise.

Improper excretion of digestive enzymes and hydrochloric acid in the stomach.

Inability to produce sufficient amount of bile and pancreatic enzymes.

Overconsumption of carbohydrate type food.

Improper eating habits such as:

> Drinking liquids with meals. Liquids dilute the stomach enzymes and acids.
>
> Eating between meals.
>
> Eating a large meal at dinner time.
>
> Eating close to bedtime.
>
> Improper food combining, which confuses the stomach.

The enzymes and acids produced to break down protein are different from those produced to break down carbohydrates. When both kinds of enzymes are produced at the same time, they can suppress each other if a person has a weakened digestive system. Weight gain can occur when food is not broken down into its smallest molecules. If food is not fully ingested into your system to be utilized as energy, it turns into fat.

Avoid eating protein and starch together. Protein with vegetables or starch with vegetables can be metabolized properly. Eat fruit two hours before or two hours after protein or starches. Unless the filling is vegetables, sandwiches made on bread are not a good food combination.

Extremely hot or cold food. These cause the stomach to contract and expand. Contraction slows down the acids and enzymes from the stomach lining, causing indigestion, and interrupts the complete cycle of digestion. Expansion causes overexcretion of acids and enzymes, creating heartburn and gas. Expansion also causes you to desire more food since your stomach becomes enlarged.

CONVENTIONAL TREATMENT

Low calorie diet.
Diet pills—amphetamines.
Balloon in stomach.
Stomach stapling.
Protein drinks.
Starch blockers.

PROBLEMS ASSOCIATED WITH CONVENTIONAL TREATMENT

A low calorie diet is not natural. Eventually you become so hungry, you cannot continue on this diet so you fail and gain back all the weight you lost and more. Furthermore, you lose lean body muscle mass which helps burn fat. In addition, heart muscle is also lost from lack of protein. A low calorie diet also adjusts your body to a lower metabolism, which interferes with further weight loss.

Diet pills speed up all bodily processes causing nervousness and anxiety, leading to undue stress on all bodily systems (endocrine, nervous, digestion, etc.), giving rise to the eventual breakdown of the entire body.

The balloon must be replaced every four months. This is a medical procedure which could be unpleasant. The balloon is made of plastic, a foreign material which can be the cause of infections and depression of the immune system and can lead to other ailments.

Stomach stapling is a very serious medical operation with a high mortality rate. It is not reversible. This procedure does not address your set point (appestat in the brain which controls satiety). In the long run, it acts only as a temporary controlling method, which is eventually overcome by the person's own appetite.

Protein drinks do not actually replace food. They are low in fiber, vitamins and minerals which the body needs to make up for the nutrients it is not getting because of dieting.

Starch blockers stop the digestion of sugar by fooling the body into thinking it is getting sugars. Your body can only be fooled so long until it reacts, readjusting to the starch blocker which then ceases to work.

ALTERNATIVE NATURAL METHOD

Acupressure. Appetite can be decreased by squeezing your ear lobes between the thumb and forefinger for 60 seconds.

Drink 6 ounces of grapefruit juice before meals. It contains the enzyme, amylase, and suppresses appetite.

Drink water between meals. It fills the stomach and helps decrease appetite.

One half-hour before a meal, take a combination of guar gum, pectin and fiber (sold in health food stores under various trade names). This expands in the stomach, taking up room, and also lowers blood sugar, decreasing appetite.

Take six 1200 mg. capsules of lecithin or two heaping tablespoons of the granules sprinkled on cereal or salad daily. Under normal circumstances, fat burns at 332 degrees. Lecithin helps burn fat at 98 degrees, which is body temperature. It also has the beneficial side effect of lowering cholesterol and triglycerides and helps produce acetylcholine for memory.

Apple cider vinegar promotes digestion. Mix it with monounsaturated safflower oil or olive oil and spices and herbs for a salad dressing.

Eat a high protein, low carbohydrate diet. A high protein diet will not cause loss of heart muscle, but a high carbohydrate diet eventually leads to cardiac muscle loss. The best foods are fish and organic poultry (white meat) without the skin. Do not eat shellfish because they are scavengers and have a higher fat content. Do not eat meat because it contains additives, herbicides, pesticides, DES, tranquilizers and arsenic. Arsenic is what gives the yellow color to non-organic chicken. Antibiotics and hormones, fed to fatten animals for human consumption, also fatten the humans.

Eat only low-fat, low-salt dairy products such as cheddar, Swiss Jarlesberg, farmer's, low-fat pot, hoop and cottage cheese and low-fat plain yogurt with active live cultures.

Do not eat fried or scrambled eggs, because high temperatures oxidize the lecithin in the yolk. The lecithin is needed to break down

the fat and cholesterol. Oxidation also causes production of free radicals. Eat only soft cooked or poached eggs.

Avocados, olives and Macademia nuts are good sources of protein
and are low in carbohydrate (sugars), but they are high in vegetable
fat.

Unlimited amounts of salad, greens and sprouts are allowed with
any other type of food, or alone.

Vegetable juices are allowed—low sodium tomato or mixed vegetable and aloe vera juice.

*Avoid the following foods which have a high carbohydrate con-
tent:*

Potatoes	Yams	Spaghetti
Beets	Carrots	Chips
Rice	Corn	Crackers
Bread	Pasta	Junk food
Milk	Fruit	Pretzels
Fruit juice	Hoagies	Pizza
Sugar	Molasses	Maple syrup
Sodas	Candy	Chocolate

*Drink the following herbal teas, which decrease appetite and aid
digestion:*

Red raspberry	Fennel	Fennugreek	Chickweed

The following amino acid also depresses appetite:

L-Phenylalanine, 500 mg. four times a day on an empty stomach.

Eat breakfast like a king and dinner like a pauper, because the
thyroid works fastest in the morning and slows as the day pro-
gresses.

Why Other Diets Are Wrong

The skin, bones, blood and bodily tissues consist of protein and
fat. Carbohydrates are energy foods. By eating fewer carbohydrates
and more protein, the body will utilize fat and protein as energy.
Protein which is not utilized will turn to fat. The body will burn its
own fat as energy if no fat from sugar is added. This is orchestrated
by the burning of ketone bodies (ketosis).

As a person gets older, the complex carbohydrate diet is improper because insulin is needed to break down the carbohydrates.

Due to the aging process, insulin production is lower, so the body tries to overproduce it, causing the blood sugar to drop too low, causing hypoglycemia (low blood sugar) which enhances the craving for sugar.

Excess insulin in the bloodstream causes an increase in appetite which makes one hungry. Insulin is used to break down carbohydrates. Thus, the more insulin in the bloodstream, the greater desire for carbohydrates, which eventually cause weight gain if they are not burned off. Proteins and fats are metabolized by the digestive enzymes.

You can eat as much of the allowed foods as you want. You must drink eight glasses of water daily, between meals, to rid the body of toxins and help with elimination of undigested foods. You may have clear soups, made without starchy vegetables, such as bouillon, clear chicken broth and tomato soup.

This diet actually burns off excess fat and has no negative effects. Since you do not eat the carbohydrates, you do not add more fat, and existing fat is converted into energy and disappears. It is safe for everyone except diabetics.

Carbohydrate restriction ketosis is different from diabetic ketosis and is not dangerous if the kidneys are working properly and the B.U.N. readings are in normal levels.

Exercise

Twenty minutes of any type of aerobic exercise will burn off excess calories faster. In addition a six block brisk walk after each meal causes less need for insulin production. High blood sugar is burned off through muscle activity.

Maintaining Ideal Weight

Gradually incorporate complex carbohydrates back into the diet, but not when eating protein. This regime can be varied every fourth day. This gives the fat-producing foods time to burn off without adding unwanted weight and causes less intolerance to allergenic foods.

Monday and Friday	Fruit or juices
Tuesday and Saturday	Bread, pasta, or spaghetti
Wednesday and Sunday	Yams, beets, or carrots
Thursday	Rice, corn, or beans

Why To Avoid Caffeine

Caffeine activates sugar into the system from glycogen stored in the liver, causing weight gain. Caffeine causes excretion of adrenalin from the adrenal glands which stimulates the release of stored sugar (glycogen) from the liver. Glycogen is converted into glucose, creating an energy lift which is similar to the ingestion of carbohydrates. Therefore, the same process takes effect, and if you do not burn off the glucose, you gain weight. Since caffeine is a diuretic, it also flushes vitamins and minerals from the kidneys.

Why To Avoid Alcohol

Alcoholic beverages before a meal raise insulin levels which increases appetite.

Osteoporosis

DEFINITION

Deterioration and thinning of bones (except in the skull). Symptoms include bones that break easily or spontaneous fractures, dowager's hump, pain in the long bones, and shrinking. The best way to determine bone density is by the dual photon densometer.

CAUSES

Menopause in women due to a decreased supply of estrogen. Women lose three percent of bone mass every year following menopause. Prior to menopause, estrogen raises copper levels, which aid calcium in bone production. The disease is more common among women and four out of five of them eventually develop some degree of osteoporosis, compared to one of five men. Fewer cases of osteoporosis are seen in overweight women because carrying extra weight strengthens bones.

The primary reason for your loss of bone mass is your inability to properly metabolize calcium through the digestive tract. Hair analysis tests reveal only fifteen percent of osteoporosis patients are deficient in calcium. Seventy-five to eighty percent demonstrated excessive amounts of calcium. This research revealed that osteoporosis can occur either from lack of calcium or an excess amount. The problem lies in the breakdown of calcium into a soluble form, allowing it to be absorbed into your system rather than stored as calcium deposits, leading to kidney stones, gallstones and arthritis.

Improper activity of the parathyroid glands, which manufacture parathormone, a hormone instrumental in regulating blood calcium levels. If these levels are low, the body will draw calcium from the bones to elevate them and thinning of the bones will occur.

Lack of exercise.

Calcium phosphorus imbalance. Ideally this should be one part phosphorus to two and a half parts calcium. Meat contains 25 times as much phosphorus as calcium. Soft drinks also contain excessive amounts of phosphorus.

Food passing through the digestive tract too rapidly prevents proper absorption of calcium. This is usually caused by hyperthyroidism.

CONVENTIONAL TREATMENT

Hormone replacement therapy for women.

Steroids.

Physical therapy

PROBLEMS ASSOCIATED WITH CONVENTIONAL TREATMENT

Hormone replacement therapy can cause cancer of the endometrium, increased risk of breast cancer, gallbladder disease and high blood pressure.

Cortisone blocks production of bone in the body and slows absorption of calcium in the intestines.

ALTERNATIVE NATURAL REMEDIES

Diet

Maintain proper calcium phosphorus balance by eliminating high phosphorus foods such as meat and soft drinks. Get more calcium derived from food. Best sources are dairy products, canned salmon and sardines with bones, dark green leafy vegetables, nuts and seeds, especially sesame seeds.

Do not eat uncooked cereals and grains as they contain large amounts of phytic acid which may inhibit calcium absorption. Uncooked greens contain oxalic acid which also inhibits calcium absorption.

Normal calcium absorption is only 20 to 30 percent of that which is ingested. Hydrochloric acid in the stomach, which is needed for calcium absorption, decreases as a person ages. Calcium absorption is also dependent on Vitamin D. However, do not drink milk with synthetic Vitamin D as it can deplete the body of magnesium. The correct balance between calcium and magnesium in the body should be one part calcium to two parts magnesium. In order to get this ratio, more magnesium than calcium must be taken.

Fat in moderate amounts moving slowly throug' the digestive tract is needed for calcium absorption.

Apple cider vinegar used as a salad dressing aids calcium absorption.

Drinking too much distilled water may cause mineral depletion. To avoid this, add one to two teaspoons of sea water (available in health food store) to each gallon of water.

Supplements

Bone Builder, a new supplement on the market contains micro-crystalline Hydroxyapatite concentrate, obtained from raw bone. It is made up of calcium, magnesium, zinc, copper, manganese, fluorapatite, silica, iron, rubidium, platinum and other micronutrients which are used by nature to build bone. Take according to directions on label.

Do not take antacids as a source of calcium since they are of the carbonate type, which is poorly absorbed. Some antacids are composed of talc, which is poisonous to the body. Antacids also slow down the digestive process.

Magnesium citrate, 1200 mg. daily.

Vitamin D, 400 to 800 I.U. daily. Some doctors have prescribed dosages up to 5000 I.U. daily for short periods of time, to reverse the weakening effects of osteoporosis.

Fluoride, in high doses, given by Holistic physician.

Vitamin C, 1000 mg. three times daily, aids in the breakdown and absorption of calcium.

Pancreatin with hydrochloric acid (digestive multiple enzyme), 1 with each meal.

High potency vitamin/mineral supplement such as VM75, 1 daily.

Do not take minerals with meals because certain foods contain blocking compounds (phytates and oxalates). Bones tend to reabsorb at night so that is the best time to take calcium.

Herbs

Horsetail strengthens bone and helps speed healing process of fractured bones.

Rue helps harden bones and teeth.

Oat straw is high in silicon and rich in calcium.

Comfrey provides proper amounts of calcium and phosphorus for strong bones.

White oak bark is high in calcium.

Black walnut contains silica.

Marshmallow is rich in calcium.

Queen of the meadow is high in Vitamin D.

Skullcap is high in calcium and magnesium.

Amino Acids

Aspartic acid, per label, is an excellent mineral carrier.

L-Histadine, per label, promotes stomach digestive secretions.

L-Lysine, 500 mg. twice daily, promotes bone formation.

L-Arginine, per label, hastens bone repair. Bones may actually heal twice as fast.

Adjunctive Methods

Exercise such as walking, swimming and light calisthenics promote strong bones. Jumping on a trampoline is one of the best exercises for osteoporosis. It provides enough impact without damaging joints.

It is important for women to bank bone from the ages of fifteen to thirty-five, since bone production is highest in this age group and decreases drastically after menopause. Therefore, high calcium intake from foods and supplements should be incorporated at this time. Calcium-depleting type foods such as sugar, alcohol, denatured food (overcooked), foods containing preservatives and chemicals and any other type of processed foods should be strictly avoided.

For your additional information, research by Dr. L.C. Kervran, called the Biological Transmutation Concept, states that calcium derived from food and supplements is not absorbed by the body in cases of osteoporosis. Bone should be strengthened by silica, potassium and magnesium since they are more effective in improving mineral metabolism.

P.M.S. AND MENSTRUAL PROBLEMS

DEFINITION

P.M.S. affects some women a week or two before their menstrual period begins. Symptoms include undue anxiety, weight gain, bloating, cramping, depression, personality changes, breast tenderness and unusual cravings. The average woman spends six years of her life in P.M.S.

CAUSES

Obesity.

High estrogen levels and low progesterone levels. When estrogen is overactive, it causes an inflammatory condition in the pelvic area. Estrogen is overproduced by smoking, a high salt diet, too much sugar consumption, an imbalance of vitamins and minerals and lack of exercise. A high dairy intake also raises estrogen levels because estrogen is given to cows and is secreted in their milk.

A drop in blood calcium and zinc levels and a rise in copper levels can cause nervousness, insomnia, depression and migraines. High estrogen raises copper levels, and copper is antagonistic to zinc.

Low thyroid function.

Exhausted adrenal function.

Decreased amounts of blood and oxygen reaching the uterus at this time is partially responsible for cramping.

An imbalance between inflammatory and anti-inflammatory prostaglandins, (PGE-1 and PGE-2).

CONVENTIONAL TREATMENT

Birth control pills.

Diuretics.

Antidepressants.

Anti-inflammatory medication.

Antispasmodics for cramping.

PROBLEMS ASSOCIATED WITH CONVENTIONAL TREATMENT

Medications address the symptoms, not the cause of the problem.

Birth control pills have side effects, including blood clots, migraine headaches, liver toxicity, heart problems, vision changes, shortness of breath, swelling of ankles and feet and breast tenderness.

Diuretics also remove other electrolytes, causing an imbalance of calcium, magnesium, potassium and sodium, which eventually affects the actions of the thyroid and adrenal glands.

Anti-inflammatory drugs deplete calcium, cause stomach ulcers, water retention and psychosis.

Antidepressants have the potential to become addictive. Doses originally given become ineffective and more has to be taken for the desired result.

ALTERNATIVE NATURAL REMEDIES

Diet

Eliminate all unnatural, denatured, processed foods such as cookies, cake, candy, chocolate, white flour, sugar, ice cream, molasses, maple syrup, honey, potato chips, pretzels, fried foods, overly-cooked foods, caffeine (in coffee, soda, cocoa and medicine), pizza, hoagies, fast food, alcohol, wine and beer.

Eat natural type foods including whole grains such as barley, oats, wheat, millet, brown rice, couscous and kasha. Protein should come from fish, organic white meat of chicken and turkey without the skin and plain non-fat yogurt.

If overweight, go on a weight reducing diet.

Avoid foods that produce estrogen such as soy beans, fats, sugars, carrots and yams (except for wild Mexican yams).

Avoid foods containing folic acid and PABA which stimulate estrogen production. They are legumes, endive, oats, wheat germ, alfalfa, brewer's yeast, sunflower seeds and liver.

Avoid all foods from animals that have been given hormones. Eat poultry and meat from organic sources only.

Foods to stimulate the thyroid are potatoes, apples, mushrooms, sesame seeds and kelp.

To raise progesterone levels, eat wild Mexican Yams. Progesterone buffers estrogen levels and helps clear the uterus.

Supplements

Vitamin B6, 250 mg. twice daily, acts as a diuretic.

Magnesium citrate, 400 mg. three times daily, improves glucose tolerance, reduces craving for sweets, helps slow heavy menstrual bleeding and relieves muscle spasms.

Vitamin B6 and magnesium work together to reduce estrogen and increase progesterone levels. They also make the body more acid. During the part of the cycle when the body is high in estrogen, it is too alkaline.

Vitamin A from fish liver oil, 25,000 I.U. twice daily, and from Beta carotene, 25,000 I.U. twice daily, reduce P.M.S. symptoms.

Vitamin E, 400 I.U. twice daily (build up slowly), reduces breast symptoms and increases circulation of blood carrying oxygen to the uterus. It also assists Vitamin A storage and utilization.

Omega 6 fatty acids (GLA) from Evening Primrose oil, 6 capsules daily, or from borage oil 240, 3 capsules daily, helps produce pro-staglandin PGE 1, needed for anti-inflammatory purposes. Prostaglandin PGE 1 helps alleviate painful uterine spasms and inhibits glucose in-duced insulin secretions which specifically reduces sugar cravings.

Fish oils, omega 3 fatty acids, 2 capsules three times daily.

Vitamin C, 1000 mg. three times daily, acts as a natural diuretic and overall antioxidant.

Calcium citrate, 500 mg. twice daily.

Vitamin B12 sublingual, 500 mg. three times daily, helps alleviate nervous disorders.

Zinc picolinate, 30 mg. twice daily, helps move vitamin A from the liver to the bloodstream and stimulates the immune system.

Iron, 18 mg. twice daily, helps prevent anemia from blood loss. It should be organic. Use iron fumerate or gluconate, not iron sulfate. When inorganic iron and Vitamin E are taken at the same time, they counteract each other. Take Vitamin E and iron eight hours apart.

Inositol, 500 mg. twice daily, and

Choline, 500 mg. twice daily, helps to enhance liver function to break down the active estrogen.

Vitamin B1, thiamine, 100 mg. twice daily, stimulates the thyroid and relieves muscle cramping.

Thyro-Vital by Ethical Nutrients stimulates the thyroid.

Note: Several P.M.S. combinations are available in Health Food Stores. If using combinations in lieu of, or with, above supple-ments, be careful not to double dose. Check labels carefully.

Herbs

Bayberry for uterine bleeding.

Wild yam alleviates uterine cramps and produces progesterone which is imbalanced (if it is too low in relation to estrogen).

Black cohash contains natural estrogen and can be used in place of synthetic estrogen. Natural estrogen is not as inflammatory as synthetic (conjugated estrogen).

Blessed thistle helps balance hormones.

White oak bark.

Dong Quai is the queen of all herbs for women. It has a tranquilizing effect on the central nervous system and nourishes female glands.

Squaw vine helps strengthen the uterus.

Amaranth reduces excessive menstruation.

Golden seal promotes hormone harmony, but do not take it if you have any blood sugar irregularities. Do not take this herb more than ten days at a time without a three day break.

Sarsaparilla contains progesterone.

Cramp bark is not only a uterine sedative, but also relaxes the ovaries.

Chasteberry.

Amino Acids

L-Methionine, 500 mg. twice daily on an empty stomach, reduces estrogen to estradiol, a less active type of estrogen.

Adjunctive Remedies

Sitz baths.

Massage therapy.

Acupressure.

Note: Thinner females store less estrogen, decreasing the effects of P.M.S. Some female athletes and marathon runners produce such small amounts of estrogen that they go to the other extreme and do not menstruate at all. This can be an even worse situation than having P.M.S.

PARKINSON'S DISEASE

DEFINITION

A progressive form of neurological degeneration causing the destruction of an important type of nerve cell. Symptoms are cramping, muscle rigidity, staring facial expression, drooling, speech impairment, walking with a shuffling movement, weight loss and diminished appetite. Many patients perform a pill-rolling movement, utilizing the thumb and forefinger which rub against each other constantly.

CAUSES

An imbalance of chemicals in the brain, notably dopamine and acetylcholine. These two neurotransmitters act as message transferring chemicals between the nerve cells (neurons) that coordinate muscle function.

Heavy metal toxicity. Aluminum, cadmium, arsenic, lead and mercury have a tendency to slow the energy-producing area of the cells in the section of the brain that controls muscular activity. These heavy metals must be chelated out of the body by means of chelation therapy or D-Penicillamine, an oral chelator. Aluminum is found in cookware, baking powder, commercial salt, antiperspirants, antacids, foil wrap, drinking water, medicines and toothpaste.

Manganese miners in Peru had a high degree of Parkinson's Disease due to low dopamine. Manganese is antagonistic to dopamine.

CONVENTIONAL TREATMENT

Replenishing of the neurotransmitter L-Dopa (levadopa).

PROBLEMS ASSOCIATED WITH CONVENTIONAL TREATMENT

Replenishment of L-Dopa does not address the initial cause of the deficiency and eventually the continual use of L-Dopa atrophies the body's natural ability to produce any amount of dopamine. This means you'll be dependent on this medication for the rest of your life.

Medicines all have side effects because they do not allow the body to produce its own defenses. When the body manufactures its own medicine, it works on a feedback system that recognizes when enough has been produced. Then it automatically ceases generating that chemical and utilizes just what is necessary. Synthetic drugs are not affected by the feedback system, so they build up to such a high degree as to cause an overload, with side effects in the body.

ALTERNATIVE NATURAL REMEDIES

Diet

A high complex carbohydrate, low protein diet will supply the higher amount of glucose needed to nourish the brain area that has been depleted of energy.

Eat whole grains such as barley, oats, wheat, millet, brown rice, couscous and kasha.

Best fruits are apples, pears, stone fruits, strawberries and cherries.

Eat more salads, greens, broccoli, sprouts, asparagus, spinach, cabbage, carrot tops, dandelion, turnip and collard greens, potatoes, beets, yams, carrots, beans, peas, lentils and corn.

Protein should be from tofu, hummus (chick peas), tahini (sesame seeds) and seitan. Cut back to extremely small amounts of protein originating from animals.

Drink lots of distilled water and mixed vegetable juices.

Supplements

Vitamin B complex, 100 mg. twice daily, as an enhancer of the brain/nervous system. Note: if taking L-Dopa, do not take extra B6 because it slows its assimilation. However, if B6 is given as part of combined B vitamins along with magnesium, the condition will improve.

Zinc picolinate, 30 mg. twice daily, prevents B6 from interfering with L-Dopa.

Magnesium citrate, 400 mg. three times daily. A deficiency of this mineral causes a deficiency of brain dopamine.

Calcium citrate, 500 mg. twice daily, is good for the transmission of nerve impulses.

Vitamin C, 1000 mg. three times daily.

Vitamin E, 200 I.U. daily for first week. Build up slowly to 800 I.U. Latest investigations of Vitamin E therapy in Parkinson's Disease show high amounts (up to 30,000 I.U.) have highly beneficial results. This must be done under the care of a holistic physician only.

Octocosanol, 2 mg. three times daily, for muscle control.

CoEnzyme Q10, 30 mg. three times daily

Vitamin B12, sublingual, 500 mcg. twice daily.

Herbs

Damiana has stimulating properties and is useful for nervousness.

Skullcap gives immediate relief of chronic and acute disease stemming from nervous afflictions.

Amino Acids

Phenylalanine, 500 mg. three times daily on empty stomach, acts as a nerve stimulator.

L-Tyrosene, 500 mg. three times daily on empty stomach, for mood regulating.

L-Tryptophan, 500 mg. three times daily on empty stomach, is a calming neurotransmitter. (Be sure to obtain from pure sources.)

L-Methionine, per label.

GABA, per label, for brain metabolism, and relaxes neurons.

Theonine, 500 mg. twice daily on empty stomach.

Adjunctive Remedies

New types of cranial electrical stimulating devices have been investigated and may stimulate the degenerative electrical vibrations in the neurons. One such device is manufactured by Liss Co. located in Northern New Jersey.

A new diagnostic procedure B.E.A.M. (Brain Electrical Activity Mapping) can pinpoint the area of the brain which is deficient in brain rhythms. With this knowledge, that area can be reintroduced to the neurotransmitter that is lacking.

PROSTATE ENLARGEMENT

DEFINITION

The prostate is a walnut-size organ, part muscle and part gland, that surrounds the male urethra at the base of the bladder. It secretes semen, a milky fluid that is ejected with the sperm. The urethra is the canal from the bladder to the exterior of the body. When the prostate enlarges, it squeezes the urethra, diminishing the flow of urine. In extreme cases it can stop the flow. It also exerts pressure on the bladder, causing the feeling of having to urinate when the bladder is actually empty. The prostate enlarges in most men, starting approximately at age thirty-five, unless a proper nutritional problem is practiced.

Two important diagnostic procedures to be sure the prostate is not cancerous are:

Prostatic acid phosphatase (male pap test).

Prostate specific antigen.

A transurethral biopsy can miss nodes on the outside of the gland. A transurethral ultra sound test is more effective.

CAUSES

Lack of nutrients. Clogged arteries slow circulation to your prostate, depriving it of the nutrients it needs. Therefore, it enlarges to compensate for those nutrients that are not available.

Poor circulation.

High fever. Fever indicates the presence of a bacterial or viral infection. Fighting the bacteria or virus depresses the immune system. If the immune system is not working at 100 percent capacity, all parts of the body tend to work at abnormal rates. If the prostate is already slightly enlarged, it would enlarge even more so.

Atherosclerosis—Plaque formation. This slows circulation of blood to the tiny capillaries in the prostate, depriving its tissues of full amounts of nutrients (vitamins, minerals and oxygen). Therefore, the prostate does not work at its optimal capacity.

Arteriosclerosis—Hardening. The arteries and capillaries feeding the prostate become hardened and crack like a garden hose left out in freezing weather. This causes leakage of blood, preventing it from reaching the tissues to nourish them.

CONVENTIONAL THERAPY

Surgery

Prostatectomy—Removal of the prostate.

T.U.R.—Transurethral resection. The inner core of the prostate is scrapped away. Nowadays this procedure may be done with a laser.

Hormonal Therapy

Reduction of testosterone, the male hormone, by Lupron or Fludimide.

PROBLEMS ASSOCIATED WITH CONVENTIONAL TREATMENT

Surgery. The side effects from surgery can lead to problems from scar tissue later on in life. Scar tissue tightens up and shrinks, causing pressure on the surrounding areas which will eventually cause their malfunction. Furthermore, bacteria is attracted to scar tissue because it is dead tissue.

Side effects of surgery are weakening of your immune system, and the possibility of contracting other diseases or infections in the hospital. Anesthesia can cause brain malfunction leading to dementia problems in the future.

Hormonal therapy treats your symptoms rather than their cause and has a rebound effect when it is stopped, resulting in even more enlargement of your prostate. Hormonal treatment for prostate enlargement can cause blood clots.

ALTERNATIVE NATURAL REMEDIES

Diet

While the prostate is enlarged, it is important to avoid all sugar or sugary type food and all fruit and fruit juices. Sugar displaces oxygen in the bloodstream, slowing down the supply of oxygen to the prostate tissues. When sugar is present in the bloodstream, the body becomes acidic, causing destruction of nerves. These nerves are needed to send messages regarding the proper feeding of tissues back and forth to them.

Supplements

Wheat germ oil capsules, two to three times a day.

Chelated zinc, 50 mg. three times a day, until shrinkage occurs.

Manganese, 50 mg. three times a day, until shrinkage of the prostate occurs.

Vitamin C, 1000 mg. three times daily.
Beta carotene, 25,000 I.U. twice daily.
Vitamin E, 400 units three times a day.

Herbs

Saw palmetto berries (herbal capsules), 3 times a day.

Amino Acids

GABA (Gamma aminobutyric acid), 500 mg. twice daily on empty stomach, moderates smooth muscle response in the genito-urinary tract.

Prostech, a combination of three amino acids—glysine, glutamic acid and alanine, per label.

Most supplements should be taken on an empty stomach when possible so the vitamins, minerals and amino acids will not compete with the nutrients from the meal. The body in its infinite wisdom absorbs natural nutrients from food first and will not get enough of the additional nutrients that are needed therapeutically.

Adjunctive Remedies

Localized Hypothermia

Raising the temperature of the prostate causes shrinkage of the cells. (This procedure is done in the doctor's office.)

Take sitz baths. Sit in water as hot as you can tolerate for 30 minutes 4 times a day.

Most of the time nutritional supplements and sitz baths will work. If they do not, an electrode can be implanted in the prostate to raise its temperature. This procedure is performed by a urologist.

Prevent enlarged prostate

Ejaculate at least two times a week. The method is unimportant and can depend upon circumstances and the individual's personal preferences. This prevents semen from stagnating in the prostate.

Don't hold back ejaculation. Maintaining an erection for an over-long period of time does not necessarily make you a great lover. It causes pressure on the prostate cells, and they rupture. Refer to books such as *The Joy Of Sex*.

Exercise to increase the mobility of the prostate. Lie flat on your back and touch the soles of the feet to each other. Pull the feet to the groin slowly. Then kick out the legs. Do this exercise 10 times twice daily.

Self massage. Insert a lubricated finger (you can wear a latex finger guard) into the rectum and massage. You have to go in 2 to 3 inches and rub toward the front of the body to reach the prostate.

Take one third the therapeutic dose of suggested supplements for maintenance.

Limit coffee, spicy foods, alcohol and smoking which all constrict arteries and capillaries, slowing the circulatory process to the prostate and causing more inflammation.

SHINGLES (HERPES ZOSTER)

DEFINITION

A painful viral infection of the central nervous system, characterized by the eruption of blisters on the skin above the nerve paths. This usually occurs on the upper torso, neck or face, along the path of the trigeminal nerve, but can occur on other parts of the body. The condition can last up to three months and can lead to post herpetic neuralgia. If blisters appear anywhere near the eye area, see an ophthalmologist immediately, as blindness could result if the cornea gets affected.

CAUSES

A deficiency in the immune system reactivates the dormant chicken pox virus.

CONVENTIONAL TREATMENT

Painkillers.

Anti-inflammatory drugs.

Vitamin B12 injections.

PROBLEMS ASSOCIATED WITH CONVENTIONAL TREATMENT

Medication addresses symptoms rather than causes and has side effects.

Painkillers have the propensity to become addictive, as patients take increasingly larger doses for them to remain effective. Medications that contain acetaminophen will actually prolong the illness.

Anti-inflammatory drugs depress the immune system, deplete calcium, cause stomach ulcers, water retention, psychosis, dizziness, nausea, headache, constipation, diarrhea and vomiting.

ALTERNATIVE NATURAL REMEDIES

Diet

Eliminate all unnatural, denatured, processed foods such as cookies, cake, candy, chocolate, white flour, sugar, ice cream, molasses, maple syrup, honey, potato chips, pretzels, fried foods, overly-cooked foods, caffeine (in coffee, soda and medicine), pizza, hoagies, fast food, alcohol, wine and beer. Do not eat vitamin enriched cereals containing inorganic iron which exacerbates herpes zoster.

Eat natural type foods, including whole grains such as barley, oats, wheat, millet, brown rice, couscous and kasha. Protein should come from fish, organic white meat of chicken and turkey without the skin and plain non-fat yogurt.

Yogurt and buttermilk not only help alleviate pain, but prevent extension of the lesions and promote healing.

Supplements

Vitamin B12, sublingual, 500 mcg. twice daily, helps reduce pain. (It is more effective if injected by physician.)

Vitamin C, Ester C, 1 gram every hour until lesions dry. High amounts of C may cause diarrhea. If this occurs, cut back. Be sure to use buffered C in these dosages. It would be more effective if given intravenously or by injection, and usually relieves symptoms in three to four days. Intravenous Vitamin C does not pass through the intestines so more can be given with less diarrhea. Do not take Vitamin C with inorganic iron since the combination can inactivate Vitamin E.

Vitamin E, 1200 to 1600 I.U. daily. Work up slowly to this dosage, and continue for at least six months. This also aids in controlling post herpatic neuralgia.

Magnesium citrate, 400 mg. four times daily.

B complex, 100 mg. twice daily.

Vitamin B6, 200 mg. twice daily.

Vitamin A, fish liver, 25,000 I.U. once daily (four weeks only).

Vitamin A, Beta carotene, 25,000 I.U. four times daily.

Zinc picolinate, 50 mg. twice daily (three weeks only).

Omega 3 fish oil, 2 capsules, three times daily.

Borage oil, 240, 1 three times daily.

Bromelain, 500 mg. twice daily between meals, acts as an anti-inflammatory.

The following three medicines relieve symptoms and pain. They must be administered by a holistic physician.

AMP (adenosine-mono-phosphate).

Colchicine.

Mexital.

Herbs

Horehound, apply topically.

Myrrh soothes inflammation and speeds the healing process.

Oregon grape acts as a blood cleanser.

Slippery elm bark, helps assist activity of the adrenal glands which help produce the body's own anti-inflammatory, cortisone.

Cayenne red pepper for pain.

Amino Acids

L-Lysine, 500 mg. four times daily on empty stomach, helps fight the herpes virus.

L-Tryptophan from pure sources, as a calmative.

Note: Stay away from argenine-producing foods such as soybeans, peanuts, nuts, pork, turkey and chocolate, since they tend to deplete the body of lysine which is needed to control the herpes virus.

Adjunctive Remedies

Vitamin E oil or aloe vera gel can be applied topically to ease the pain. Also, try rubbing the inside of a banana skin on the eruption. A chemical in the banana skin acts as an anti-inflammatory.

Zostrex (capsicum-cayenne red pepper extract) cream has been found beneficial for pain relief of eruptions.

SKIN CONDITIONS
(ECZEMA, PSORIASIS, SEBORRHEA, ACNE ROSACEA)

DEFINITION

Eczema is an inflammatory reaction to a variety of stimuli from outside and within the body causing swelling, redness, blistering and weeping on the skin. The skin becomes thickened and scaly with intense itching.

Psoriasis is the overproliferation of the outer layer of skin cells. These cells usually take 19 to 21 days to form and slough off. In patients with psoriasis, this cycle is shortened to a 3 to 4 day period, causing such a high degree of proliferation, production and sloughing of skin that there is a chronic condition of red scaly patches. Immature cells do not have enough time to mature and constantly accumulate as dead debris.

Seborrhea is an excessive increase in the sebum secreted by the sebaceous glands causing benign lesions that can occur anywhere on the skin or the scalp. It is also a condition where cells proliferate at a faster than normal rate and are sloughed off as scales. Sebum, which accumulates in the area of the hair follicles, solidifies, causing hair loss, dandruff and other scalp problems.

Acne rosacea usually occurs on the nose and cheeks and is characterized by pustules, red papules and dilated blood vessels. Enlargement of the nose can occur. It is also called W.C. Fields nose. He was an actor and comedian in the 1920s and 30s.

CAUSES

The basic cause of these skin conditions is an overabundance of toxic materials that should be eliminated from the body via the kidneys, liver, bowel and lungs. An overabundance of toxic materials overloads your kidneys, liver, bowel, and lungs and is forced to exit through your skin as bacteria. It then mixes with sebaceous oil, blocks your sebaceous glands and causes a buildup of bacteria on your skin, leading to cell destruction and an inflammatory condition.

A genetic predisposition, which means, if one is born with the specific gene for a skin condition and activates that gene by abusing the body, the ailment may develop.

Allergic reactions to food, environmental abuses, medicine, the sun, clothing, perfumes, cosmetics, shampoos, soaps and laundry detergents.

Alcohol, smoking, spicy foods and caffeine cause dilation of the capillaries which could exacerbate the condition.

Overly dry skin from lack of humidity, especially from forced hot air heat.

CONVENTIONAL TREATMENT

Corticosteroid drugs applied topically.

Moisturizing creams.

Antihistamines for itching.

Ultraviolet light therapy for psoriasis.

Coal tar ointments and shampoos.

Preparations containing salicylic acid, zinc pyrithione and selenium sulfide.

Retin A.

Acutane.

Antimetabolite medication to prevent excessive proliferation of epidermal cells by interfering with division of the cells.

Psoralen (PUVA), a medication taken internally, followed two hours later by exposure to long wave ultraviolet light on the lesions. The medication is released from the body via the skin in two hours, and the ultraviolet light photoactivates the area, causing it to bind with the DNA and slow overproduction of immature skin cells.

PROBLEMS ASSOCIATED WITH CONVENTIONAL TREATMENT

Anything applied to the skin is absorbed by the system. In these conditions, large areas of skin are affected and large amounts of medication are used. Since these medications are of a synthetic nature, they must be eliminated by a weakened liver, causing additional damage to it.

Steroids cause an increased risk of heart attack, stroke, liver changes, hair loss and breast enlargement. They can cause skin damage if overused or applied to the wrong areas.

Moisturizers do not address the cause. They are only palliative.

Antihistamines cause drowsiness and even more dryness.

Coal tar is messy and time consuming. Relapses usually occur, and these products can stain light hair.

Antimetabolites' effects are not limited to the skin. They also interfere with metabolism of all body cells, specifically the bone marrow and the gastrointestinal tract. One of these drugs, methotraxate, is also prescribed as a chemotherapy agent for cancer patients. Its side effects are nausea, vomiting, sore mouth, liver, blood and bone marrow problems.

PUVA has been known to increase the possibility of skin cancer.

Retin A often causes reddening and dryness of the skin and increased photosensitivity.

ALTERNATIVE NATURAL REMEDIES

Diet

Food allergies must be addressed. Most skin conditions are simply a side effect of eating foods that are not fully metabolized, which then become an enemy of the body, causing a histamine release leading to skin irritation.

The diet should consist of all natural type foods. Eat fruits, vegetables, whole grains, brown rice, complex carbohydrates, organic fish, chicken and turkey, yogurt, cheeses, soft cooked or poached eggs and low fat soups. Drink at least eight glasses of distilled water daily. Use lots of garlic which acts as a natural antibiotic. Sunflower seeds are good for dry skin.

If digestive problems, such as burping, heartburn, flatulence or indigestion are present, they should be addressed because they are an indicator that food is not being digested properly. Food that is not assimilated normally, produces an overabundance of toxic materials which may pervade the body through the skin.

Avoid all sugars, processed foods, white flour, chemicals, preservatives, coloring agents, fried foods, caffeine and alcohol.

Supplements

Pancreatic enzyme with hydrochloric acid, 1 or 2 with each meal.

Fish oil (omega 3 fatty acids), 2000 mg. three times daily.

Borage oil (240), 1 three times daily, helps convert lineolic acid to anti-inflammatory prostaglandin E1.

Folic acid, 800 mcg. four times daily, helps regulate red blood cell folate levels which allows the necessary nutrients to reach the skin.

Vitamin A, fish liver, 25,000 I.U. twice daily, and Vitamin A, Beta carotene, 25,000 I.U. four times daily, help regulate skin proliferation.

Selenium, 200 mcg. twice daily, aids in activating glutathione per-oxidase, which slows the formation of inflammatory antibodies (leukotrines).

Zinc picolinate, 50 mg. twice daily, aids in the healing process of the skin, helps metabolize Vitamin A through the liver and aids tissue respiration.

Mucopolysaccharides, per label, acts as an anti-inflammatory agent and energizes weak cells.

A good multi-vitamin/mineral combination such as VM75, one daily.

Vitamin C, 1000 mg. three times daily.

Vitamin E, 400 I.U., one daily.

Psorex, per label, is an excellent supplement for the skin. It is derived from fumeric acid, a known rehabilitator for degenerative cells in the skin.

Herbs

Birch, applied topically, contains birch oil which softens dry skin.

Burdock acts as a blood cleanser and removes toxins.

Dulse is high in iodine for thyroid regulation.

Kelp helps regulate the thyroid which is essential for skin regeneration.

Squaw vine helps kidney function.

Gum weed is useful for all skin disorders.

Jojoba aids in the removal of impregnated sebum and lowers the ph of the scalp to a healthier, more acidic condition.

Horsetail (silica) tones the skin.

Rosemary stimulates the skin.

Sage is a good scalp tonic.

Oregon grape (barberry) eliminates toxins.

Amino Acids

L-Proline, 500 mg. once daily on empty stomach, helps maintain elasticity of the skin.

L-Taurine, 500 mg. twice daily on empty stomach, helps control psoriasis.

L-Cystine, 500 mg. once daily on empty stomach, aids in skin formation.

Adjunctive Remedies

The water in the dead sea and the air in the region aid the healing process of inflammatory skin conditions.

Adriatic mud relieves psoriasis.

Sea water baths (available in health food stores).

One-half cup of apple cider vinegar added to a tub of water aids in restoring acidity to the skin. Restoration of healthy skin is dependent on maintaining a proper acid, alkaline balance.

Do not bathe too frequently and limit use of soap. Try to obtain low ph (acid type) soap.

AED cream with lanolin and aloe vera gel or cream are soothing to irritated skin.

Rub the inside of a banana skin on inflamed areas of the skin. It works wonders and has been used for thousands of years.

Emotional and nervous disorders must be addressed. The immune system will be compromised unless the patients change their negative attitude toward life. Negative attitudes cause tightness in the body leading to slowdown of the organs' production of the body's beneficial chemicals.

THYROID PROBLEMS
(OVER OR UNDERACTIVE THYROID)

DEFINITION

The function of the thyroid gland is to supply thyroxin, the thyroid hormone, to individual cells for the purpose of metabolism. Oxygen is utilized in this procedure. The oxygen content is regulated in the cells by thyroxine. When insufficient oxygen is supplied, the patient is a slow oxidizer and hypothyroidism, (underactive thyroid) occurs. If an overabundance of oxygen is supplied, the patient is a fast oxidizer and has hyperthyroidism (an overactive thyroid).

Insufficient thyroxin thickens blood, causing clotting which can lead to heart attacks. An overabundance of thyroxin thins blood and can cause hemorrhaging.

Another name for hyperthyroidism is Grave's Disease. An autoimmune condition known as Hashimoto's disease sometimes causes an underactive or overactive thyroid.

Symptoms of hyperthyroidism are extreme nervousness, anxiety, protruding eyes, excessive perspiration, high body heat, extreme hunger, rapid pulse and loss of hair. Goiter (a morbid enlargement of the thyroid gland) can occur from the overproduction of thyroxin. When any organ is overworked, it will enlarge.

Symptoms of hypothyroidism are fatigue, dry skin and hair, low body temperature, mental sluggishness, lower intellectual capacity and goiter. Dark circles under the eyes may indicate low thyroid. Any organ in the body which perceives itself as not supplying the full amount of its specific chemical, will enlarge itself in an effort to utilize the enlarged area for production of that chemical.

Two types of nodules may appear on the thyroid. "Hot" nodules mean the area is still functional and not dangerous. "Cold" nodules imply that the area is dysfunctional and could be malignant, although cancer of the thyroid is rare.

CAUSES

A dysfunction of the pituitary gland can cause a deficiency or overproduction of the thyroid stimulating hormone. A decreased amount of thyroxin in the thyroid causes a slowing of metabolism and slower burning of calories. An overproduction of thyroxin leads to a more rapid burning of calories.

A deficiency of nutrients that supply the thyroid with ingredients needed to perpetuate its normal function. These nutrients are iodine, tyrosine and Vitamin B1.

An attack by the body's own antibodies on the thyroid tissue causing destruction of thyroid cells (an autoimmune disease).

Radiation therapy for enlarged or infected tonsils and enlarged adenoids destroyed the thyroid. This form of treatment was discontinued in the early 1950s.

Fast oxidizers are deficient in magnesium.

Too much calcium slows the thyroid.

Too much potassium speeds up the thyroid.

Copper reduces high potassium levels lowering thyroid function.

CONVENTIONAL TREATMENT

Hypothyroidism is treated by replacing the missing hormone with levothyroxine (a synthetic thyroid).

Hyperthyroidism is treated surgically, with methimazole, an anti-thyroid medicine, or radioactive iodine (I31).

PROBLEMS ASSOCIATED WITH CONVENTIONAL TREATMENT

If the dosage of levothyroxine is not calculated exactly, the problem can continue or even reverse. Side effects are digestive problems, headache, nervousness, hand tremors, rapid or irregular heartbeat, shortness of breath, skin rashes and bone loss.

When the thyroid is removed surgically, patients must take synthetic thyroid for the rest of their lives.

Methimazole's side effects are numbness, loss of taste, dizziness, skin rash and tingling of fingers.

Anti-thyroid medications may contain yellow dye #5, which has caused allergies in humans and cancer in rats.

Radioactive iodine can destroy too much thyroid tissue or may not burn out enough. You must be on medication for the rest of your life.

ALTERNATIVE NATURAL REMEDIES

Diet

Iodine from kelp, seaweed, sea salt and fish balance thyroid function.

Foods with thio-oxazidone block iodine absorption. Patients with underactive thyroids should not eat them. These foods should be incorporated into the diet of people with overactive thyroids. Thio-oxazidone is found in raw spinach, lettuce, cabbage, turnips, beets and rutabaga. It is inactivated by cooking these vegetables.

Soybeans and products made from them, such as tofu, contain a thyroid depressing element and should be consumed by those with overactive thyroids and eliminated from the diet of patients with underactive thyroids.

Eight ounces of pumpkin seeds supply 1250 mg. of L-Tryptophan, a calming neurotransmitter.

A word of caution. Regular iodized salt contains dextrose (sugar), which is used to remove the purple color of iodine. Sodium bicarbonate is added to oxidize iodine. Sodium silica aluminate is also added to aid in pouring. Sugar and two extra types of sodium have been added to this salt. Use only sea salt.

Supplements

Hyperthyroids should take the following supplements:

Copper, 4 mg.

Multi-vitamin/mineral combination such as VM75.

Vitamin A fish liver oil, 25,000 I.U. once daily.

Vitamin A Beta carotene, 25,000 I.U. twice daily.

Vitamin E, 1200 I.U. (work up to this dose slowly).

Iodine (in the form of kelp), 4 mg.

Vitamin C, 1000 mg. three times daily.

Zinc picolinate, 30 mg. twice daily.

Calcium citrate, 600 mg. twice daily.

Lithium, per label. (A natural form is available in health food stores.)

Hypothyroids should take the following supplements:

Multi-vitamin/mineral combination, such as VM75.

Vitamin B1, 100 mg. three times daily.

Vitamin C, 1000 mg. three times daily.

Vitamin E, 400 I.U.

Potassium, 1000 mg.

Zinc picolinate, 30 mg. twice daily.

Magnesium citrate, 400 mg. three times daily.

Do not take extra supplemental calcium as it slows the thyroid.

Herbs

Irish moss is high in iodine and is useful to balance both hyper and hypothyroidism.

Black walnut is a natural source of iodine.

Watercress regulates metabolism.

The following two herbs are useful for hypothyroids:

Parsley is high in potassium.

Sarsaparilla stimulates the metabolic rate.

Amino Acids

L-Tyrosine, 500 mg. four times daily on an empty stomach, is a precursor of thyroid hormone and is good for balancing the system.

L-Lysine, 500 mg. twice daily on empty stomach, reduces the inflammatory response of antibodies (for autoimmune response).

An effective natural-type thyroid replacement is Armor Thyroid. It is a natural ingredient and must be prescribed by a physician.

TINNITUS

DEFINITION

Abnormal sounds in the inner ear such as ringing, thumping, buzzing, roaring or hissing.

CAUSES

Injury to head.

Inner ear infection.

Too much fluid which causes pressure.

Backup in Eustachian tubes.

Aspirin or salicylate type medication.

Low blood sugar.

Dysfunction of minute nerve endings in the ear.

Antibiotics.

High fats in the diet which cause red blood cells to accumulate and stick together, thickening the blood.

Reduced flow of blood to the inner ear.

Heavy metal toxicity.

Food allergies.

Deficiency in Vitamin A and/or a deficiency in the B vitamins, which are both important for nerve function.

Overproduction of adrenalin from stressful situations which causes a decreased blood supply to the inner ear.

An imbalance in the electrolytes which control fluids in the inner ear.

Loud noises from airplanes, rock concerts, explosions, pneumatic drill hammers, gunfire, etc.

CONVENTIONAL TREATMENT

At this time, the orthodoxy has very little to offer for the treatment of tinnitus. They often suggest that the patient seek psychotherapy.

ALTERNATIVE NATURAL REMEDIES

Diet

Eliminate sugar, processed foods, artificial foods and fats.

Test for food allergies. In order to learn if you are allergic to a specific food, stop eating that food for four days. Take your pulse, and then eat that food by itself. Wait 20 minutes and check the pulse again If it goes up or down 10 points or more, a food allergy may be present. Cytotoxic testing is an accurate blood test, performed by a physician for food allergies.

Supplements

Multi-vitamin/mineral such as VM75, one daily.

Vitamin B complex, 100 mg. once daily, to help improve nerve function. (Some Vitamin B complex is in VM75, but more is needed, especially niacin which aids circulation.)

Vitamin A, fish liver oil, 25,000 I.U. once daily.

Vitamin A, Beta carotene, 25,000 I.U. twice daily.

Phosphatidyl choline, per label, to break down fats.

Niacin, 200 mg. three times daily, thins blood and widens arteries for better circulation.

Chromium picolinate, 200 mg. three times daily, to alleviate low blood sugar.

CoEnzyme Q10, 30 mg. twice daily, is a cell stimulant.

DMG, 125 mg. once daily, is an oxygen facilitator.

Germanium, 50 mg. twice daily, is an oxygen facilitator.

Omega 3 EPA, 2000 mg. three times daily, aids circulation and stops clumping of platelets.

Herbs

Ginseng aids all hearing activity.

Angelica aids hearing.

Plantain clears your inner ears of mucous.

Capsicum, (cayenne red pepper) improves circulation in your ears.

Ginger improves circulation of ears.

Amino Acids

L-Taurine, 500 mg. three times daily on empty stomach, helps alleviate low blood sugar.

L-Histadine, per label, improves function of your auditory nerve.

Adjunctive Remedies

Recent investigations have shown antihistamines may help alleviate tinnitus, but they do have side effects such as drowsiness and drying of tissues.

Using a hearing aid may alleviate tinnitus.

Hair analysis should be done to uncover mineral deficiencies and heavy metal toxicity.

Hydrogen peroxide, 35 percent food grade, per label (not 3 1/2 percent sold as antiseptic), contains an extra atom of oxygen and aids oxygen flow to inner ear. Or apply hydrogen peroxide gel to the soles of the feet.

Investigate tinnitus support groups in your area. They usually have the latest information available for your specific problem.

ULCERS

DEFINITION

An inflammatory condition in the lining of the stomach and/or duodenum causing pain and burning when the stomach is empty or while food is being digested. The esophagus may also be an ulcer site. Ulcers have a tendency to bleed. Blood would be observed in the stool as being dark in color. Ulcers can cause hemorrhaging to the point where a person could bleed to death.

CAUSES

Improper food combining.

Overproduction of hydrochloric acid from the stomach which may erode the mucous-protected stomach lining. Mucous consistency may not be sufficient to protect the lining from erosion.

Latest scientific studies have shown a certain bacteria, campylobacter, has been found in the stomach which may lead to ulcers.

Overproduction of the enzyme, pepsin, may also cause ulcers.

Overingestion of alcohol, tobacco, aspirin, anti-inflammatories and spicy foods irritate the stomach lining.

Not chewing properly. Chewing mixes food with saliva, a digestive enzyme.

CONVENTIONAL TREATMENT

Bland diet while inflammatory process is present.

Antacids.

Surgery

Cutting of the vagus nerve to decrease stomach acid.

Drugs such as Cimetidine, Zantac and Carafate.

Diagnostic procedures such as upper GI series and endoscopy.

PROBLEMS ASSOCIATED WITH CONVENTIONAL TREATMENT

A bland diet is deficient in fiber necessary to activate peristalsis, the automatic contractions that propel food through the digestive system. Fiber is also necessary for regular bowel movements.

People over 40 are often deficient in hydrochloric acid and pepsin. Therefore, taking antacids is counterproductive since not enough acid is being produced to process food.

Surgery addresses only symptoms, not causes, and years later, scar tissue in the stomach area from surgery can lead to problems.

Eventually no digestive acids are produced after severing the vagus nerve. This leads to serious problems digesting food.

Cimetidine and Zantac work by blocking the release of stomach acids. This causes problems digesting protein and fatty type foods which can lead to difficulties in assimilation of the fat soluble vitamins, A, E, D and K. Other adverse effects of these drugs are confusion, sore throat, irregular heartbeat, constipation and skin rash. Side effects of Carafate are constipation, dizziness, dry mouth and skin rash.

If you are given a GI series, you will receive a large amount of radiation from the X-ray, which causes destruction of the DNA of the chromosomes of cells. This may lead to cancer later in life.

ALTERNATIVE NATURAL REMEDIES

Diet

Eliminate foods which increase acidity such as coffee, processed sugars and white flour. If ulcers are active, avoid cereals, whole grains and nuts. Avoid sour fruits such as citrus, pineapple, strawberries, pomegranate, tomato, sour apples, grapes, peaches and plums. Sweet fruits are acceptable and include bananas, dates, figs, raisins, Thompson and muscat grapes, prunes, sun dried pears and persimmons.

The diet should be high in fiber.

Eat small meals six times daily rather than three large meals.

Avoid foods that are too hot or too cold. Try to ingest food at body temperature.

Never fast with an ulcer condition.

Potato juice and cabbage juice (Vitamin U) accelerate the healing process.

Eliminate fried foods and heated oils.

Try not to eat raw fruits and vegetables since they are difficult to break down.

Eliminate processed sugary-type foods and sugars which stimulate insulin production. Insulin may be destructive to cells in the stomach lining.

Ulcers are caused by an excess of acid. The patients should be treated with alkalizing food such as cooked vegetables, sweet fruits, buckwheat, millet, coconut, sprouted grains and seeds. Avoid acid-producing foods such as dairy products, meats, flour products, sweets, eggs, fats and grains until the condition subsides.

Eat fruit separately from other foods. Do not combine protein and starches at the same meal. As food journeys through the pyloric valve (the exit from the stomach to the duodenum), the valve becomes confused if partially digested proteins and carbohydrates are present at the same time. The valve is designed to open two to three hours after ingestion of proteins and fats and one to one and a half hours following consumption of carbohydrates. If proteins and carbohydrates arrive at the same time, the pyloric valve may allow undigested proteins out of the stomach too soon, or it may not open, retaining the carbohydrates, which will then ferment and cause gas.

Until the condition subsides, do not consume foods containing calcium, such as dairy products, which promote secretion of gastrin, a digestive hormone that releases acid to the stomach. Previously the orthodoxy, in their infinite wisdom, used milk and cream as neutralizing agents in the stomach, when in reality they exacerbated the condition.

Drink distilled water which helps ease pain.

Supplements

Vitamin E, 1000 I.U. (work up slowly to this dosage) is an antioxidant which helps slow down inflammatory conditions.

Pantothene, 300 mg. three times daily, is an anti-inflammatory.

Zinc picolinate, 50 mg. twice daily, is very important for healing of ulcers.

Vitamin C, buffered only (ester C), 1000 mg. three times daily, helps in the healing process.

Vitamin/mineral combination such as VM75, one daily.

Vitamin A, fish liver oil, 25,000 I.U. once daily, and

Vitamin A, Beta carotene, 25,000 I.U. four times daily, aid in tissue repair.

Quercetin (bioflavanoid), 500 mg. three times daily.

Aloe vera gel, 2 ounces three times daily (keep in refrigerator). This is the most successful treatment for ulcers. It stands head and shoulders above any anti-ulcer medicines. It binds to pepsin in the stomach and blocks hydrochloric acid from the parietal cells. It also increases enzyme activity and cellular metabolism. People who are squeamish about swallowing the gel, can take four glasses of aloe vera juice daily.

Acidophilus, 2 billion or more viable cells each capsule, four times daily, restores ratio of bacteria.

Under no circumstances should ulcer patients take any type of digestive enzyme.

Herbs

Peppermint oil aids healing in inflammatory conditions.

Deglycyrrhizinated licorice improves mucous in the digestive tract, and aids in the healing of inflamed tissue.

Cayenne red pepper aids digestion and stimulates blood flow to the area, promoting healing.

Chickweed helps digest fatty substances and aids in helpful production of stomach mucous.

Plantain helps normalize stomach secretions and neutralize stomach acids.

White oak bark helps alleviate internal bleeding, cleanses mucous membranes and repairs damaged tissues in the stomach.

Golden seal alleviates internal bleeding.

Myrrh aids inflammatory conditions and speeds healing.

Slippery elm bark has anti-inflammatory properties.

Amino Acids

L-Arginine, 1000 mg. three times daily on empty stomach, promotes healing of ulcers.

L-Glutamine, 500 mg. four times daily, acts as an antacid. (Natural antacids do not work the same as synthetic antacids, which stop all production of acids.)

L-Glycine, 500 mg. three times daily, acts as an antacid.

L-Histadine, per label, reduces histamine production. The overproduction of histamine into the stomach may trigger acid secretions.

Adjunctive Remedies

Stop smoking, as it stops the natural bicarbonate produced from the pancreas which acts as a natural antacid in the body. Smoking also stimulates release of glucose from the liver, raising insulin levels which exacerbate the ulcer condition in the stomach.

There is a new theory that bacterial infection may cause ulcers. Natural antibiotics are echinacea, garlic, golden seal and bee propolis.

Avoid stress and try to relax. Acids in the stomach are activated by preparation for digestion. This activation can also be caused by stress-related activity, which produces a rise in adrenalin, activating stomach acids. When this occurs and there is no food entering the stomach, these acids have nothing to digest and start to devour the stomach lining. Therefore it would be wise for ulcer patients to have something in their stomachs at all times so this process does not occur.

Mucous which is formed on the stomach lining is there for protection of the tissues. In certain individuals, this mucous is lessened, causing a higher susceptibility to erosion of the lining. Thus the original stress factors, whether they are environmental, psychological, philosophical, dietary or medicinal, must be addressed. Under these circumstances, therapy in progress to alleviate the ulcerative condition will not be effective because the stress factor is the dominant reason for the original condition.

VARICOSE VEINS

DEFINITION

Venous blood (in the veins) which returns to the heart via the veins, is not actually pumped back by the heart. Blood is ejected from the heart through the arterial system to all parts of the body. As this blood returns through the veins, it is pushed forward by muscle contraction and expansion.

Inch by inch, the blood works its way up the extremities and eventually back to the heart and lungs for oxygenation and renewed distribution. A series of valves is built into the veins. As an area fills with blood, the valve beneath it closes and the one above opens. The blood is forced up into the next area by muscle undulation.

With varicose veins, the valves actually leak, slowly allowing the blood to pool in a lower chamber, causing swelling of the vein, characterized as visible bluish cords in the legs.

Symptoms of varicose veins are:

Pain in the legs.

A heavy feeling in the legs.

Swelling of foot or ankle.

Leg cramps while sleeping.

Change in skin color.

Rash on the legs.

CAUSES

An individual can have a genetic predisposition to weak valves or weak veins.

Injury to the area.

Thrombophlebitis can damage the valves and walls of the veins.

Pregnancy.

Overweight.

Tumors.

Tight clothing, especially elastic topped stockings.

Aging, which causes loss of muscle support and elasticity in the area.

Prolonged standing or sitting lead to diminished circulation.

Constipation puts pressure on the leg veins.

Prolonged sitting on the toilet cuts off circulation from the back of the legs.

CONVENTIONAL TREATMENT

Elastic stockings, which force blood into deeper veins.

Scleratherapy which is the injection of a solution to obliterate a section of the vein.

Surgery—stripping of the veins.

When an area is obliterated either surgically or by injection, the surface veins are the ones that are treated. The greater saphenous vein, which is the inner vein, takes over circulation in the legs.

Vasodilators.

Blood thinners.

PROBLEMS ASSOCIATED WITH CONVENTIONAL TREATMENT

Elastic stockings must be expertly fitted in order to put pressure on the correct areas.

The patient may be allergic to the material injected into the veins. Scleratherapy has a high failure rate and may cause permanent brown pigment stains on your skin.

Side effects of surgery are weakening of your immune system from anesthesia and the possibility of contracting other diseases or infections in the hospital.

Vasodilators raise blood pressure which may then overtax an already weakened heart.

If patients on blood thinners are not properly monitored, the blood may become too thin, leading to hemorrhage and death.

ALTERNATIVE NATURAL REMEDIES

Diet

Obese patients must lose weight. The best diet is one high in protein and low in carbohydrate. See chapter on obesity.

Eliminate fats and sugars which thicken your blood and cause undue pressure on the valves in the veins.

Eat a diet high in fiber to prevent constipation. Include whole grains, bran, fruit with skin, vegetables, beans, complex carbohydrate tubers (root vegetables, nuts and seeds).

High levels of cholesterol and triglycerides thicken the blood, putting undue stress on the valves in the veins. These levels must be brought down. Refer to chapter on cholesterol.

Supplements

Vitamin/mineral combination such as VM75, one daily.

Vitamin E, 1200 I.U. (work up to this dose slowly), acts as a blood thinner and keeps platelets from adhering to each other so they won't clump together and therefore swell your veins.

Rutin (bioflavanoid), 200 mg. three times daily, and

Quercetin (bioflavanoid), 500 mg. three times daily, aids healing, prevents bruising and strengthens your capillary walls.

Pycnogonal (bioflavanoid), per label.

Shark cartilage, per label, is an anti-inflammatory and also prevents new growth of arteries which could lead to more inflammation.

Bromelin, 500 mg. twice daily between meals, is an anti-inflammatory.

Fish oil, 2000 mg. three times daily, acts as a blood thinner and anti-inflammatory.

Borage oil 240, 1 three times daily, produces prostaglandin PGE1, an anti-inflammatory.

Garlic, 500 mg. four times daily, an anti-inflammatory and blood thinner.

Vitamin A, Beta carotene, 25,000 I.U. twice daily, and

Vitamin A, fish liver oil, 25,000 I.U. once daily, aid in the repair of endothelial cells and stimulate the immune system.

Niacin, 200 mg. twice daily, acts as a vasodilator and blood thinner.

Vitamin C, 1000 mg. three times daily, aids in the assimilation of minerals, nourishes the capillaries and stimulates the immune response.

Herbs

Rue strengthens your capillaries and veins. It also contains large amounts of rutin.

White oak bark aids repair of damaged tissues.

Capsicum for circulation.

Prickley ash increases circulation throughout the body.

Mistletoe aids the circulatory system.

Horseradish is good for circulation.

Ginger stimulates circulation.

Cloves increase circulation.

Horse chestnut is an anti-inflammatory.

Amino Acids

L-Histadine, 500 mg. twice daily, acts as a vasodilator.

L-Proline, per label, helps promote growth of muscles, tendons and ligaments.

Adjunctive Remedies

Walking, swimming and cycling all aid lower body circulation.

Lie on a slant board with head lower than feet and do leg lifts.

Avoid sitting for prolonged periods. People with desk jobs should not sit for more than 30 minutes at a time.

Do not sit on the toilet too long.

If bedridden, wear elastic hose.

Elevate foot of bed four inches.

Rub castor oil into inflamed areas twice daily.

Do not cross legs.

Take cool showers rather than hot baths.

YEAST INFECTIONS
(SYSTEMIC CANDIDA)

DEFINITION

A systemic disease caused by the overproliferation of yeast (single cell fungi producing rhizodes which are long root-like structures). This usually occurs in the lower intestines and colon, causing an imbalance in the bacterial flora of the area. Under normal conditions, yeast is kept in check by the immune system. When the yeasts proliferate to a high enough degree to imbalance the good bacteria, the disease is incorporated into the system. It is not a localized disease. It is a disease of the entire body.

When out of control, the yeasts have the ability to bore through and produce leakage in the lower intestine and colon, allowing undigested food and toxins to proliferate into the bloodstream where they are carried to other parts of the body to do their damage. Although these toxic reactions can develop in any part of the system, they occur most often in the vagina (vaginitis), tongue and upper esophagus (thrush), the feet (athlete's foot), the fingernails and toenails.

As yeast dies off, it emits a toxic substance that poisons the body (Herksheimer's syndrome).

The same deficiencies in the system that lead to candida (lack of oxygen in the cell) can also lead to cancer.

Yeast can change its surface to resemble a white blood cell and the antibodies will pass it by (antigenic). It can also resemble hormones and give false signals.

CAUSES

Antibiotics, prednisone and birth control pills deplete the good bacteria, allowing the bad bacteria (yeast) to proliferate.

Dietary infractions, such as high sugar intake, too many dairy products, fruits, fermented foods, vinegar, pickles, tofu, foods containing yeast such as most breads, beer and wine.

Sluggish digestion. Transit time for food should be twelve to eighteen hours. A longer transit time is an invitation for candida.

Heavy growth of candida on the mucosa of the intestines slows the absorption of nutrients such as vitamins, minerals and amino acids, depressing the immune system which is needed to defend the body against disease.

The overproliferation of parasites in the lower intestine (pinworm, tapeworm, hookworm, roundworm or ringworm) should be addressed for the complete treatment of candida. Stool test may not be conclusive. Patient must be tested by swabbing the inner wall of the intestine.

Excess zinc (over 150 mg.daily) promotes growth of candida and suppresses the immune system.

Molds in cheeses.

Yeast infections proliferate in an alkaline environment. During pregnancy, sugar stores in vaginal cells and increases their alkalinity. Susceptibility is also higher during menstruation since the vaginal area is in a more alkaline state at that time. Most P.M.S. formulas, which include B6, magnesium, calcium and Evening primrose oil, acidify the vaginal and uterine areas. In a more acid condition, they are better able to destroy negative yeast proliferation.

Tampons and diaphragms left in place too long.

The string from the I.U.D. breeds bacteria.

Vaginal yeast infections can be sexually transmitted.

Cyclosporins used to depress the immune system during organ transplants.

CONVENTIONAL TREATMENT

Systemic candida is not recognized by orthodox medicine as an ongoing disease. Therefore they do not have a satisfactory treatment. They treat candida as a fungal infection using nystatin, keloconazole and clotrimazole. Sites of involvement are treated locally with antifungal ointments and powders.

PROBLEMS ASSOCIATED WITH CONVENTIONAL TREATMENT

Orthodox doctors do not treat through diet, which is crucial in the treatment of the disease, nor do they attempt to strengthen the immune system. Thus the condition is never eradicated. By addressing only the symptoms, the underlying native disease remains dormant and will erupt and spread throughout your body again.

Antifungals may interact with other medications, and they also can cause digestive upsets. Oral doses of nystatin prescribed for vaginitis are ineffective because nystatin is not absorbed into the body. Therefore it does not travel to the vagina. Nystatin is derived from mold, a substance causing allergic reactions in many people, and its base is made from acorn syrup, which is basically sugar.

ALTERNATIVE NATURAL REMEDIES

Diet

Eliminate all sugars and foods containing sugar, tea, coffee, fruit juices, fruits, dairy products, beer, wine, alcohol, processed or smoked meats, tofu, mushrooms, packaged foods, fermented foods and anything made with baker's yeast. Brewer's yeast is not harmful.

Eat meat and poultry from organic sources only. Animals raised for commercial purposes are fed antibiotics and steroids. When these are ingested, they cause the overproliferation of negative bacteria.

Eat whole grains, brown rice, oats, barley, nuts, seeds, fresh vegetables, bread without yeast, organic eggs, fish and meat. Quinoa (pronounced keenwa) and amaranth are two grains that are excellent sources of protein.

Specific anti-candida foods are garlic, onions, ginger, cabbage, broccoli, barley, yogurt, wheat germ and olive oil.

Try not to exceed 60 to 80 grams of carbohydrates daily. The number of grams of carbohydrates in the allowed foods are:

Brown rice, one cup	152
Tomato	7
Potato	25
Onion	14
Beets, one cup	13
Lettuce, one cup	1
Beans, one cup	40
Almonds, one cup	27
Walnuts, one cup	15
Peanuts, one cup	29
Peanut butter, 1 tbsp.	3
Alfalfa sprouts, one cup	0
Lentil sprouts, one cup	0
Sunflower seeds, one cup	29

Supplements

Germanium, 100 mg. three times daily, acts as an oxygen facilitator, and candida cannot live in an oxygen environment.

Vitamin B15 (DMG), 125 mg. twice daily, enhances the immune system and acts as an oxygen facilitator.

Dioxychlor, administered by a holistic physician, acts as an anti-oxidant against fungi. (It is an oxygenator.)

Capryllic acid, per label, to destroy candida fungi.

SOD (superoxide dismutase), per label, is an enzyme that flushes excess residue from the body (free radicals and superoxides).

CoEnzyme Q10, 30 mg. three times daily, stimulates the immune system and enhances cell energy.

Vitamin A, Beta carotene, 25,000 I.U. four times daily, and

Vitamin A, fish liver oil, 25,000 I.U. once daily, help repair the surface of the endothelium.

Hydrogen peroxide, 35 percent food grade, 3 drops three times daily the first day. Work up to 25 drops three times daily by day 16, and then gradually decrease the dosage. Always take antioxidants with hydrogen peroxide because of the extra production of free radicals. This should only be taken while under the care of a holistic physician. This may cause stomach upset. If it does, use hydrogen peroxide gel applied to the soles of the feet. This method bypasses the digestive system. For more information on hydrogen peroxide, write to Vital Health Products, Ltd. Box 164 Muskego, Wisconsin 53150.

Vitamin C, 1000 mg. three times daily.

Multi-vitamin/mineral combination such as VM75, one daily.

Vitamin E, 800 I.U. Build up to this dosage slowly.

Magnesium citrate, 400 mg. three times daily.

Calcium citrate, 500 mg. twice daily.

Vitamin B6, 100 mg. three times daily.

This combination of magnesium, calcium and B6 is useful to acidify the alkaline condition that occurs during menstruation.

Acidophilus, enteric coated, each capsule containing 2 billion or more viable cells, four times daily.

Essential fatty acids, either Evening primrose oil, 1 capsule six times daily, borage oil (240), 1 capsule three times daily, flaxseed oil, per label, or linseed oil, per label. These convert to gamma linolenic acid which converts to anti-inflammatory prostaglandin PGE1, which counteracts the effects of inflammatory prostaglandin PGE2 and leukotrienes.

Biotin, 2 mg. twice daily.

Chlorophyll, per label, relieves itching and burning and has the ability to break down poisonous carbon dioxide. It inhibits growth of this anaerobic bacteria and releases free oxygen.

Shark cartilage, 12 capsules daily for three weeks. Then gradually decrease the dose. This is an anti-inflammatory.

Pancreatic enzymes, 2 between meals three times daily, eliminates dead yeast from the body.

Herbs

Garlic, enteric coated, 500 mg. four times daily, is a potent antifungal agent.

Sage counteracts yeast infections.

Wintergreen.

Pau D'Arco (double the amount on the label) counteracts candida and stimulates immune response.

Australian tea tree oil fights bacteria and fungi.

Black walnut hulls alleviate parasites.

Buckthorn alleviates parasites.

Pumpkin seeds alleviate parasites.

Echinacia aids in the production of interferon and is a T-cell stimulator, which enhances the immune system.

Feverfew acts as an anti-inflammatory.

Amino Acids

L-Glutathione, 500 mg. twice daily on empty stomach, acts as an antioxidant, destroys free radicals, and stimulates the immune system.

L-Histadine, 500 mg. twice daily, reduces the release of leukotrines.

L-Glutamine, 500 mg. four times daily on empty stomach, promotes regeneration of intestinal mucosa.

Adjunctive Remedies

Wheat grass juice contains high amounts of chlorophyll, which resemble the molecules of red blood cells, enhancing the blood supply.

Liver cleanse. Do not eat anything after noon. At 7 p.m., take 4 tablespoons of olive oil followed by 2 tablespoons of fresh lemon juice. Repeat every 15 minutes until 8:45. You will have used 16 ounces of olive oil and the juice of 12 lemons. Go to bed at 10 p.m. and sleep on right side.

If a serious illness requires the use of antibiotics, it is better to have them administered by injection instead of orally. This avoids having them pass through the intestinal tract.

The immune system must be stimulated. This is done by taking high amounts of antioxidants and changing one's lifestyle. Avoid smoking, drinking, processed foods and sugary foods. Try to avoid stressful situations. The best methods of coping with stress are biofeedback and meditation. In order for it to be effective, meditation must be practiced daily. People who think they don't have the time should realize that 15 or 20 minutes meditating twice a day takes less time than traveling to and waiting in the doctor's office, costs less and is more effective.

Meditation decreases the production of adrenalin from the adrenal glands. The overproduction of adrenalin eventually exhausts the adrenal glands, leading to a malfunction of other organs that depend on the adrenals for their activation. It also causes spasms of the coronary arteries, preventing sufficient oxygen from reaching the heart muscle.

To relieve vaginal yeast infections, douche with one teaspoon acidophilus powder and one teaspoon of apple cider vinegar in two cups of warm distilled water twice daily.

Mercury must be eliminated from the system by removing amalgam fillings which are 52 percent mercury. This must be done by a dentist fully educated in the proper procedure. Otherwise the patient's condition will be exacerbated.

Other heavy metals, such as lead, aluminum, cadmium and arsenic must also be eliminated. This can be done by two methods: chelation therapy or oral chelators, such as high doses of Vitamin C, N-Aceytl cysteine and D-Pennicilimine (prescribed by holistic physician).

For relief of parasites take Paramicociden, Artemesid Annua or Parscan. These can be purchased in any health food establishment.

EXCERPTS FROM LECTURES

WHY VITAMIN C DOES NOT CAUSE STONES

Forces against alternative natural remedies express views stating that high doses of Vitamin C cause kidney stones, because it turns into oxalic acid. The following technical information scientifically refutes their statement.

Vitamin C gives up electrons, and that is why it is a free radical scavenger. Free radicals are misplaced electrons that cause damage to cells.

It makes urine more acidic, which makes oxalic acid more soluble.

It is a mild diuretic and will wash out stones.

Calcium oxalate stones tend to deposit around nitisi of infected dead cells and bacteria. Since C is a urinary tract disinfectant, it cleans up the urine, eliminating the dead cells and bacteria, thus preventing stone formation.

C is metabolized into calcium ascorbate in the body, which makes it unavailable to oxalate.

No scientific study has ever proved that kidney stones are from Vitamin C.

THE TRUTH ABOUT L-TRYPTOPHAN

L-Tryptophan is a very effective antidepressant, calms excitory neurotransmitters, eliminates physical pain, depresses appetite and is good for insomnia.

In November of 1989, certain batches of L-Tryptophan were found to be contaminated, causing eosinophilia myalgia, an immune response problem which causes disease. The F.D.A. took all tryptophan off the market, stating it was the cause of eosinophilia myalgia. In reality, a Japanese company that produced tryptophan had not cleaned the filtering system used to eliminate the type of bacteria that caused the disease. Although it was proved that it was the contaminant rather than the tryptophan that caused the disease, the F.D.A. still did not permit it to be returned to the shelves of the health food stores. Yet, when Tylenol was found to be contaminated and caused some deaths, it was removed from the market temporarily. It is now back on the shelves of the stores. In this case a double standard is being used because Tryptophan is not allowed back on the shelves of the health food stores.

Tryptophan is found in many foods including chicken, turkey, milk and cheese. Pumpkin seeds contain 1250 mg. of tryptophan per cup. If tryptophan were the culprit, anyone eating large quantities of these foods would contract the disease, but this has not occurred. Only those individuals who took the contaminated capsules became sick. Some mail order companies are able to supply 5 hydroxy tryptophan, the next chemical pathway, which is even more effective.

ASPIRIN CAN BE BAD FOR YOUR HEALTH

The F.D.A., in their infinite wisdom, has removed tryptophan from the market, and they are constantly trying to undermine and control the entire health food industry. Yet, anyone, even a child, can go into any drugstore or supermarket and buy any amount of aspirin.

People take aspirin for any minor ache or pain. When two no longer work, they take three or four. Eventually they start taking stronger combinations, also sold over the counter. When these compounds cause ulceration in their stomachs, their doctors put them on ulcer medication, which eventually damages their livers and practically stops all production of acid in the stomach, which is needed for digestion. Without good liver function, they are more susceptible to infections, and their doctors prescribe penicillin. If they are lucky, all they get is a yeast infection. Before too much time elapses, the kidneys are damaged. If dialysis is too much of a bother, there is always the option of a kidney transplant. Then the anti-rejection drugs damage the immune system.

WHAT YOU SHOULD KNOW ABOUT THE MEDICINE YOU'RE TAKING

Antibiotics alter the uptake of glucose, cholesterol, sodium, potassium, calcium, iron, Carotene and B12. Fruit juices interfere with the absorption of antibiotics. Calcium in milk or other food blocks tetracycline.

Anticonvulsant medication can cause bone disease.

Digitalis depresses appetite.

Antacids with aluminum make phosphorus hard to absorb and make the gastrointestinal tract more alkaline, which interferes with folic acid absorption.

Mineral oil blocks nutrients A, D, E and K.

Aspirin increases the excretion of Vitamin C.

Broccoli, beef liver, cabbage, asparagus and spinach may make anti-clotting medication inactive.

Patients on MAO inhibitors must avoid foods rich in tyramine such as aged cheese, avocados, bananas, soy sauce and chicken livers. The combination can make blood pressure skyrocket and can also cause headaches.

Vitamin B6 works against L-Dopa.

Antifungal medications are better absorbed with fat.

HOSPITALS

Upon entering a hospital, patients relinquish all rights for fair treatment. They become automatons and must obey every command or suffer the consequences of falling out of favor with the powers in charge. Besides taking away your identity, what they feed you will insure a return visit.

The A.M.A. advocates that dietary fat and protein should be no more than 30 percent. Hospitals that were investigated were found to serve patients 34 to 44 percent total amounts of fat and protein.

Cholesterol should be 300 mg. daily. Lowest amounts found were 350 mg. to 532 mg.

Calcium intake should be 1200 mg. Amounts ranged from 451 to 1050 mg.

Sodium should be no more than 2500 mg. Amounts were 2605 to 3430 mg.

Fiber—20 to 25 grams advocated. Hospitals gave patients 6.5 to 8.5 grams.

5 percent of patients are in the hospital at any given time because of a medication error.

5 percent will leave the hospital with a condition they did not have when they entered.

10 percent will develop some type of infection.

3 percent will be given the wrong medicine.

HAIR ANALYSIS

Hair analysis is a valuable adjunctive procedure to uncover certain deficiencies in the biochemistry of the body. An astute hair analysis will disclose the amounts of toxic heavy metals in the system, such as lead, cadmium, arsenic, aluminum and mercury. It will also show mineral and vitamin deficiencies. Mineral ratios are extremely important to determine if certain glands are working efficiently. The two most important glands involved in the production of energy are the thyroid and adrenal glands. Proper calcium/potassium ratio is needed for the efficient operation of the thyroid. Proper sodium/magnesium ratio is needed for the adrenals.

POWER LINES

A higher than normal cancer rate has been found in areas surrounding power lines and transformers located on electric poles. This is due to the high electromagnetic fields generated by them. It has also been discovered that the IQ of children living in those areas is markedly lower than average.

Electromagnetic force fields tend to change the electric polarity of the molecule in the cells in the body, causing them to give up oxygen. This loss of oxygen lessens the energy produced in the cell. When this loss of oxygen occurs, glucose combines with less oxygen, causing the cells to become less efficient, produce less energy and eventually become diseased and dysfunctional. These cells tend to become anaerobic (without oxygen) instead of aerobic (with oxygen), the normal state of the cell. This leads to disease and dysfunctional cells.

The diseased cells form tumors because they do not divide as they should. Instead of dividing, they double continually and eventually grow ino a tumor. An analogy is doubling a penny every day for a month. At the end of the month, you would have over a million dollars. In essence, the doubling cells become a large mass, impinging on or eroding glands or organs where they reside. This is cancer.

UNDERSTANDING RECOMMENDED DIETARY ALLOWANCES

The A.M.A. says the diet should consist of:

20 percent protein.

10 percent fat.

70 percent complex carbohydrates.

In order to maintain its present weight, a body requires 14 calories per pound. A 100 pound person needs 1400 calories daily in order not to lose or gain weight. To determine how much protein to eat, take 20 percent of the total allowed calories or 280 calories from protein. 10 percent fat equals 140 calories. 70 percent carbohydrates equals 980 calories. Food composition charts, available in health food stores, show how much food equals these amounts.

LIFE EXPECTANCY

The statement that life expectancy has increased to age 73 for men and 76 for women is just a manipulation of statistics. In reality, life expectancy has remained the same for the past 2000 years. Although we are led to believe we live longer than previous populations, the difference is with improvements in diet, sanitary conditions, health care, decreased infant mortality and environmental factors. Our generation has escaped the ravages of diseases that killed people by the age of 40 to 45.

In the past, those who lived to age 45 without contracting the diseases, had a better chance of reaching their 70's than people do today because of healthier food, air and water. Those who did live that long had a better quality of life and did not spend their twilight years in nursing homes. The reason is that only the strong were able to escape the ravages of the diseases prevalent in those times, and they went on to have a happy and productive old age.

THOSE WHO SURVIVE

When a physician tells the average American he or she has cancer and only a limited time to live, the patient immediately goes into shock, loses control and is left at the mercy of the medical bureaucracy. They take their medicine and die on time, implementing a self-fulfilling prophecy.

The treatment options will be surgery, radiation, chemotherapy or a combination of the three. When chemotherapy was given to healthy volunteers in tests, most became violently ill and several died. Radiation has been shown to destroy chromosomal activity in the cells, causing deterioration and eventually illness. Radiation therapy to a specific area causes fibrosis in the surrounding tissues and damages surrounding glands and organs. The fibrous tissue becomes insensitive to chemotherapy, yet they continue to administer it. Scar tissue from surgery causes tissue degeneration in the area years later (if the patient lives that long).

Patients are told these modalities are their only choice, and they have no option but to have therapy that statistics show has failed.

People who undergo this therapy are of the mind set that physicians can do no wrong, and that whatever is advocated by conventional practitioners is best for them. These patients are not necessarily the survivors and are lucky if they survive five years. Some may not feel so lucky if the quality of their life has been diminished.

Patients opting for alternative therapy are considered mavericks even though they are a stronger set of people than their counterparts. Some alternative modalities are:

Live cell therapy.

Hyperthermia.

Supplement therapy.

Diet therapy.

Immune therapy.

Metabolic therapy.

Ozone therapy (oxygen).

WHAT YOU SHOULD KNOW ABOUT CORTISONE

Cortisone inhibits the growth of collagen (the material that holds your body together).

Cortisone actually lowers your blood supply to injured tendons.

Cortisone causes adrenal glands to shrink.

Cortisone inhibits the body from producing enough protein. (Increase your protein intake if taking cortisone.)

Cortisone decreases immunity.

Cortisone increases your craving for sweets.

Cortisone causes water retention,

Cortisone causes blurred vision.

Cortisone causes insomnia.

UNNECESSARY DANGEROUS PROCEDURES

Every year:

10,000 people die from antibiotic reactions.

2.6 million unnecessary surgeries are performed.

11,900 people die from complications of unnecessary surgery.

350,000 unnecessary radical mastectomies and hysterectomies are performed.

500,000 unnecessary tonsillectomies are performed.

300,000 unnecessary appendectomies are performed.

200,000 unnecessary coronary bypasses are performed. This procedure has been shown to be contraindicated and dangerous 80 percent of the time. It has as high as a 15 percent mortality rate in patients over 60, who die on the operating table or shortly thereafter.

30 percent of people who enter hospitals do so because of iatrogenic (doctor-caused) or drug-induced disease.

WHY NATURAL SUPPLEMENTS ARE NECESSARY

People on medication (about 125 million at any given time) develop clinical nutritional deficiencies as a side effect of prescription drugs.

95 million people are dieting improperly.

P.M.S. sufferers are deficient in iron from bleeding, calcium and magnesium causing cramping, and Vitamin B6 causing bloating.

The 54 million smokers each lose 25 mg. of Vitamin C per cigarette.

40 million people have gastrointestinal problems causing malabsorption of nutrients.

The elderly lose calcium from their bones.

The diet of most teenagers is atrocious and highly deficient.

25 million alcoholics are deficient in Vitamin A, Zinc, Magnesium, Vitamin B1 and selenium.

Birth control pills cause a deficiency of Vitamin B6 and zinc.

8,500,000 strict vegetarians are deficient in Vitamin B12, Vitamin D and specific amino acids. Phytates and oxalates in raw grains and vegetables cause malabsorption of minerals and are also too alkaline.

Lactating mothers lose vitamins and minerals.

The good news is, the orthodoxy is starting to use supplements in some cases. For example, a frequently recommended amino acid, L-Cysteine, is now routinely given in hospital emergency rooms for drug overdoses.

DANGEROUS ORTHODOX PROCEDURES

DES given to prevent miscarriages causes cancer of the vagina and cervix of female offspring.

Tonsillectomies destroyed a primary immune system defense, the tonsils.

Radiation to tonsils also destroyed the thymus gland which produces T-cells and antibodies.

The original contraceptive pills contained such high amounts of estrogen that they may have caused breast cancer.

Swine flu vaccine given to the elderly actually caused the disease which was often fatal.

Oraflex and Selacryn given for high blood pressure caused liver and kidney damage and several deaths.

Merital, an antidepressant, caused severe allergic reactions and several deaths.

Suprol, a painkiller for arthritis, caused kidney damage.

Zoma, a painkiller, caused severe allergic reactions and several deaths.

Somatotropin, human growth hormone, caused several deaths.

MER, a cholesterol lowering drug, caused cataracts.

Milk therapy for ulcers has been found to be ineffective and caused more damage because high production of acid from the stomach lining was needed to digest fat and protein in the milk. This caused exacerbation of the ulcer condition.

Bland diets were the conventional treatment for diverticulitis. Now roughage, given after the inflammatory stage has subsided, has proven to be more beneficial.

Radioactive therapy for enlarged thyroid caused cancer in later years.

Encaynide and Fleckanide, two drugs for heart rhythm disturbances that were approved by the F.D.A., may have caused 3000 deaths.

The Dalkon Shield, an I.U.D., may have caused severe cases of pelvic inflammatory disease.

Too high an oxygen content in incubators may have caused blindness in premature infants.

MANIPULATING STATISTICS

A specific therapy is 5 percent effective. This means it works for 5 out of every 100 people. Later, new therapy is discovered which is 10 percent effective. This means it works for 10 out of every 100 people. Some practitioners state the new therapy gives patients 100 percent more of a chance to live. The reality is that there is only a 5 percent edge and a 95 percent failure.

MINERALS PRESENT IN SPECIFIC HERBS

Iron .... Yellow dock and Burdock
Iodine .... Kelp and Irish Moss
Calcium .... Horsetail and Nettle
Selenium............................ Horsetail and Nettle
Sulfur .... Eyebright and Nettle
Magnesium....................... Mullein and Primrose
Sodium .... Nettle and Fennel seed
Phosphorus..................... Licorice and Chickweed
Potassium .... Camomile and Fennel
Manganese .... Peppermint and Parsley
Fluorine .... Garlic and Watercress

BENEFITS OF RAW FOOD

Foods consumed in the raw state contain enzymes that aid in the breakdown of that specific food. The stomach secretes enzymes from its lining to aid digestion. Enzymes are destroyed in food that is cooked or highly processed with chemicals. Thus the amount of enzymes in the stomach is deficient for the digestive process, leading to digestive problems and malabsorption of important nutrients. The best foods for enzymes are bananas, avocados, mangos and sprouts.

LEGAL DRUG PUSHERS

Drugs previously used are considered to have been less efficient and sometimes dangerous when new ones come on the market. Patients prescribed the earlier drugs were told they were the best thing for their particular ailment at the time. Then it was demonstrated that these were dangerous and ineffective. They are switched to a new medication which is supposed to be more effective and safer, until something newer comes out. One wonders what will be said about the new medication ten years later.

SCIENTIFIC PROOF

The orthodoxy states that a treatment is not scientifically proven until it has undergone replicable laboratory testing and/or double blind studies. Their opinion of alternative therapy is that there is no scientific proof, only anecdotal evidence. Hearing this would make one believe that all procedures performed by physicians have been scientifically validated. Yet the O.T.A. (Office of Technical Assessment) report of 1987 states that 87 percent of all medical procedures have never been scientifically verified. The two largest are coronary bypass surgery and chemotherapy.

ORTHODOX VS. ALTERNATIVE TREATMENT

The majority of conventional physicians have learned the same methods, which are to treat symptoms rather than causes of disease. A holistic doctor looks at the whole person; the body (physiological), the mind (emotional) and spirit (spiritual). The latter method is more effective since illness is just the end result of the manifestation of an imbalance.

The orthodoxy gives different names for diseases. Yet, all disease is basically the same, accompanied by immobility, malaise, pain and or depression.

Bodily abuses such as smoking, drinking, drug addiction, improper diet, stress and environmental pollution cause toxins to build up in the body. These toxins must be eliminated through the kidneys (urine), the bowels (feces), the skin (perspiration) and the lungs (carbon dioxide). When these channels cannot handle the overload of toxins, they attack specific areas of the body, causing disease. The orthodoxy does not understand this premise and consequently does not investigate the causes. For example, patients suffering from depression are not asked about their diets. Yet it has been scientifically validated that depression is caused by a chemical imbalance in the brain, which is exacerbated by deficiencies in the diet. This means chemicals (neurotransmitters) needed for brain function are either inadequate or not effective enough to perform their operational duties. It would be a simple matter to perform a blood test to determine the levels of neurotransmitters in the brain. This is done by testing the platelets. If there is a deficiency, supplementation is in order. Then the brain activity could return to normal, alleviating the original problem of depression.

Instead, patients are prescribed medicine which the body is not made of, is not deficient in, does not rebuild tissue, but just acts as a blocking agent, temporarily alleviating the symptoms. All too soon the medicine becomes addictive because larger and larger amounts have to be given as the body becomes intolerant to it. Side effects start to occur which have to be treated with yet another medicine, starting a long chain of drug-related problems.

FAST FOOD RESTAURANTS

Upon entering a well known Children's Hospital, I noticed a restaurant occupied by parents visiting with their children, who were patients. These children were being treated for diseases that other hospitals were unable to manage.

One would assume that food being served in the hospital, whether from their kitchen or from an on-site restaurant, would be wholesome. However, much to my dismay, the restaurant was of the fast food type, serving greasy french fries, burgers with a high fat content, cooked on a grille that is cleaned only once daily, and milkshakes made from sugar, artificial coloring and preservatives.

Residue from burgers that could very well have turned rancid from lying in the open air remains on the grille and is picked up by the next batch. Rancidity from these bits of food gets into the body, causing the cells to break down, leading to further disease, and these children are already in a weakened condition.

French fries prepared in a deep fryer with oil become contaminated unless the oil is changed daily, but most of these restaurants just keep adding oil. Under conditions of extremely high heat, oil breaks down rapidly, causing rancidity leading to cellular destruction. Minute bits of food left in the oil may remain there for days on end and are subsequently picked up with new food.

These children have been brought to this institution to get well, but all treatments are being counteracted by their ingestion of denatured unhealthy food. A great injustice is being done to these children by not giving them the proper diet to help their bodies heal, and a great deal of therapy is in vain.

NOTHING CAN BE DONE IN THE U.S.A.

Why is it that when a doctor in the U.S.A. has no further treatment to offer a cancer patient and the patient asks about a type of therapy out of the realm of orthodoxy, the doctor states, "There are no other treatments that are of any value."? In other countries, including Germany, Australia, Canada, Mexico, Rumania and the Bahamas, many treatments are available that are not considered alternative. They are practiced daily and have a high cure rate but are not available in the U.S.A.

At least twenty different types of therapy have been proven over and over to be highly effective against cancer. The side effects are minimal. The survival rate is high. The quality of the patients' lives is better, and they have less pain. Citizens of the U.S.A. are supposed to have freedom of choice, but are forced to select only those therapies offered by the orthodoxy. The medical bureaucracy does not permit any infringement on their domination of health care.

An orthodox physician who treats patients holistically (with supplements and alternative therapy as part of a treatment plan), risks the possibility of loss of license and imprisonment. At this time there are physicians who have stepped across the line and are paying the price for putting patient welfare above the dogma of the orthodoxy.

WHY TAKE SUPPLEMENTS

Some physicians, upon learning their patients are taking supplements, say they are not necessary because food contains everything their bodies require. Unfortunately the reality is that food purchased in supermarkets, is depleted of most nutrients by the following:

Chemical fertilizers.

Early harvesting.

No crop rotation.

Improper storage.

Freezing.

Length of time from harvesting to ingesting.

Transporting food in unsanitized vehicles that previously carried chemicals or trash.

Preservatives used in markets to extend shelf life.

Improper storage in the home.

Cooking at high temperatures, which destroys most nutrients and all enzymes needed for the digestive process.

In addition, those who are deficient in hydrochloric acid and digestive enzymes are unable to assimilate what they consume.

INTIMIDATION

Patients are often coerced into having procedures because they are told that if this or that is not done, they will not survive. This is highly intimidating to a patient who is in a depressed or anxious state and does not have the wherewithal to make a correct decision. Patients rely on their physician's knowledge and accept what they are told.

Many of these procedures would not be needed if other modalities had been incorporated earlier

Utilizing such methods as dietary changes, physical therapy, stress reduction and use of supplements, in lieu of toxic medicines, gives the patient a chance to avoid harsher treatments.

Of course this does not apply to acute conditions or emergencies.

WHAT YOUR MIRROR CAN TELL YOU

Deep horizontal lines in the forehead indicate weak intestines.

Vertical lines between the eyebrows indicate a weak liver.

Swelling under the eyes can mean kidney problems or allergies.

Slanting crevices in the ear lobes warn of heart problems.

A crevice on the tip of the nose may mean a weak heart.

A horizontal crease over the top lip indicates weakened sexual organs.

QUIPS

For pain relief, take 500 mg. of L-Phenylalanine four times daily on empty stomach. It helps lessen the loss of pain-relief endorphins.

Rye bread is not a whole grain product. It contains 90 percent white flour and only 10 percent rye, and is also very high in salt. Caramel coloring is used to darken bread.

The amount of lead in the atmosphere is almost 500 times what it was in the fifteenth century.

Two thousand years ago the percentage of breathable oxygen was 39 percent. In 1900 it was 29 percent. In 1980, it was 20.4 percent. In 1989 it was 19.4 percent. Today in Gary, Indiana it is 5.5 percent.

Gefilte fish (traditional Jewish appetizer), is very unhealthy because its ingredients are derived from highly toxic fish such as carp, millet, pike and whitefish. High amounts of sugar and white flour are added. These are unrefined substances that cause the excretion of healthy nutrients.

Condoms are only 80 percent effective against AIDS, as 20 percent of the virus can get through them.

Arteriosclerosis is not just in the coronary arteries, but exists in every artery, arteriole and capillary in the body. This condition should be treated as a systemic rather than a local disease. Bypass surgery only treats the coronary arteries.

CASE HISTORIES

Aids

A 23-year-old homosexual graduate student developed a rash on his upper body, extreme tiredness, a constant fever over 100 degrees, loss of appetite, weight loss, swollen glands and night sweats. Examination and blood tests revealed he was HIV positive and had Kaposi's Sarcoma. His chances for survival were dim. The only therapy offered was AZT which he did not want to take because of its debilitating side effects. It causes dysfunction in the bone marrow that activates the red and white blood cells to fluctuate to such a degree that they cause other debilitating diseases. The already compromised immune system becomes even more depressed, leaving no hope for survival.

Treatment suggested was an immune system stimulating program consisting of a strict dietary regimen of only unprocessed complex carbohydrate type foods along with a minimum of four glasses of pure organic vegetables, juiced, daily. He also utilized high antioxidant type supplements, digestive enzymes to help metabolize the proper nutrients from the diet into his system, oxygen facilitators and ozone administered rectally to destroy viruses.

The program was extremely effective because of the patient's determination to overcome the disease. Patient's self-esteem has also increased by improving his relationships outside of the homosexual community, and he now leads a less stressful and more productive lifestyle.

ALLERGIES

A 43-year-old teacher was completely disabled by the effects of an allergic response to grass in May and June and pollen in August and September. She had undergone desensitization shots for three years at great expense. The desensitization program was effective for a short time, but then the allergies returned with a vengeance. Frustration and anxiety led her to try to discover another method to eliminate her problem.

She encountered a friend who described how effective her response was to a natural healing program and made an appointment with me. As in most cases of seasonal allergies, only one consultation was necessary. In order to desensitize her against pollen, I gave her immune system stimulants.

I recommended the following nutrients. Bee pollen granules (desensitizes patient against pollen), Quercetin and B6 (have antihistamine activity), Vitamin C for antihistamine activity and to stimulate the immune system, Ephedra (herb acts as decongestant) and Pau D'Arco and Echinacea as immune system stimulants.

In three days, 99 percent of her symptoms disappeared and she was able to return to work and enjoy a normal productive life.

ARTHRITIS

A 65-year-old domestic could not continue working due to severe arthritis in the joints of both knees. At times the immobility and pain was so severe that she could not get out of bed in the morning. She had to apply heat and massage her knees in order to have any mobility. After years of remissions and exacerbations, she decided to seek medical help. The first therapy suggested was knee joint replacement, with a recovery period of four months. Since she was the sole support of her family, she felt this was impossible.

She investigated other treatment options and was referred to me by another satisfied patient. When I saw her, at first she was apprehensive and overly cautious because my treatment sounded too simple. I explained that natural healing does not just eliminate symptoms, but it also regenerates tissue in the inflamed area, allowing a return to normal function.

The first thing she did was eliminate all foods from plants in the Nightshade family, including potatoes, tomatoes, peppers, eggplant and tobacco. These produce a poisonous solution in 75 percent of all arthritis patients, and when they are eliminated, pain is decreased and mobility returns. Other dietary restrictions were not necessary since her diet was basically healthy.

She also applied castor oil packs with steam heat to her knees for an hour twice daily. Walking in waist high water in a pool, massage and periodic acupuncture were highly effective. Since she was below normal weight, a weight loss program was unnecessary.

Nutrients recommended were Shark Cartilage and Sea Cucumber Extract (anti-inflammatories), SOD to rejuvenate the synovial fluid in the joints and rebuild cartilage. Fish oil and bromelain were also added for anti-inflammatory effects.

She now has full mobility and very little pain.

A 28-year-old tennis instructor suffered from lower back spasms so severe he was unable to work. Since he had been a patient of mine in the past, he asked me for my opinion of the problem. I suggested he see an orthopedic surgeon for blood tests and an evaluation of the lower back, but not take any medication or have any treatment.

His blood sedimentation rate was extremely high, denoting the presence of inflammation. X-rays revealed the 4th and 5th lumbar vertebrae and discs were fused with the sacrum (bat wing fusion) due to arthritic changes. The orthopedist recommended a surgical procedure which is extremely dangerous due to the proximity of the central nervous system in the area. It could have caused further pain and weakness in his legs.

I instructed him to use castor oil packs with steam heat twice daily and receive light massage treatments from a licensed therapist. All inflammatory foods in the nightshade family were eliminated. After his pain eased, he was taught specific low back exercises performed while lying flat. A weight reduction diet was not necessary. Anti-inflammatory nutrients were incorporated into his supplemental program. These included high amounts of Vitamin C to build collagen and to assimilate calcium into his system instead of having it lodge in his tissues. Shark cartilage and sea cucumber as natural anti-inflammatories, fish oil and cod liver oil as natural joint lubricators, Vitamin B1 as a muscle relaxant and DLPA as pain reliever were also included.

The patient was conscientious about following the program and within three weeks most of the pain decreased. He continued on the program, gradually increasing exercises to strengthen muscles, ligaments and tendons in the area. He has returned to teaching tennis and competing in tournaments and has full mobility and no pain.

ASTHMA

A 26-year-old male health food store clerk suffered from debilitating asthma attacks for a period of eight years. The attacks occurred more frequently during allergy season, often to the point of his not being able to breathe and becoming overly fatigued. At times hospital care was necessary. Treatment consisted of medication (theophylline) and various aerosol mechanical devices.

The problem exacerbated to such a degree that he spent some time in Arizona to test the area. He did not have any asthma attacks in Arizona, but when he returned to Pennsylvania, the problem returned and his conventional treatment gave him less relief than before.

I investigated his allergic responses which are usually the cause of asthma attacks. Environmental and food allergies were addressed. His immune system was stimulated with antioxidant type nutrients A, C, E, B complex, Selenium, Glutathione and Methionine. Stress management was incorporated since it depresses the immune system. If depressed, the immune system evokes allergic reactions causing constriction of the bronchial airways leading to asthmatic attacks. N-Aceytl Cysteine used as a mucous expectorant was effective and his breathing improved.

The patient has remained symptom free and is totally dedicated to the natural healing program.

A 22-year-old college student suffered from such exhausting asthma attacks that he was frequently rushed to emergency wards due to the inability to breathe, and was unable to continue his education. Adrenalin and other medications to relieve spasms in the lungs were administered. These relieved the symptoms but did not address the underlying problem, the allergic reaction. A pulmonary specialist referred him to a highly praised asthma center where it was determined that he was highly allergic to formaldehyde, a chemical found in rugs and wall board.

The frequent attacks and inability to lead a normal lifestyle led to depression. A patient of mine who was his friend insisted he consult me. Upon questioning him, I was appalled that none of the doctors suggested stimulating his immune system in order to correct the causative factors. I explained immune system function to him pertaining to how his antibodies caused overproduction of histamine—which attacks nerve endings in bronchial tubes and causes spasms and breathing difficulties.

My natural supplement program stimulated his immune system to such a degree that he was able to ward off the effects of the histamine. It consisted of high amounts of antioxidant type supplements Vitamins A, C, E, Beta carotene, germanium, Dimethyl glycine and other oxygen facilitators. We enhanced the transportation of oxygen and carbon dioxide in and out of his lungs. I also recommended magnesium to cut down the spastic conditions of his bronchioles.

His attacks diminished as long as he continued on the supplements, but when he did not take them, the symptoms returned. He became convinced that he had to keep taking the supplements and he improved so much that he easily finished his education.

BLOOD PRESSURE

While having his annual checkup, a 43-year-old architect showed a blood pressure reading of 165/102. For his age, normal readings are 120-140/60-95. He was asymptomatic, as are most cases of insidious high blood pressure.

If it is not controlled, high blood pressure can eventually lead to stroke or heart disease. His physician immediately prescribed a diuretic with a beta blocker. On a return visit, his blood pressure had dropped to 152/88. However, side effects of this medication had caused loss of sex drive, lethargy, high insulin levels, resulting in low blood sugar, and irregular heart beats which frightened him so much that he had to take tranquilizers.

While driving home from the doctor's office he happened to tune in to a health program on the radio. A nutritional medical doctor who had authored four books was discussing the negative effects of conventional hypertension therapy vs. the effectiveness of natural healing. He then contacted me.

The patient was extremely overweight, but much to my dismay was never put on a logical weight reducing plan. The only instructions he had were to eat less food and a balanced diet. The first thing I suggested was a high protein low carbohydrate diet which effectively reduced his weight. All sugars, alcohol, caffeine, processed foods and cigarettes were eliminated. Biofeedback methods were employed, in conjunction with meditation and imagery.

I began a program of nutritional supplementals to lower his blood pressure. I also gave him garlic, fish oil, Evening primrose oil, bromelain, Vitamin B6 (diuretic), L-Taurine (amino acid), Vitamin C (diuretic) along with magnesium, calcium and potassium to replace electrolytes lost from the original medicinal diuretic, plus an herbal combination to relieve his stress. An exercise program was also included.

After four weeks on the program and a weight loss of 16 pounds, his blood pressure dropped to 132/83. All previous side effects disappeared and his outlook on life changed from pessimism to optimism. Note: Natural healing nutrients will stabilize blood pressure at a normal level and not continue to lower it to abnormally low levels.

Leslie R., a 43-year-old mother of three was overweight and had high blood pressure accompanied by an irregular heart beat. Her family doctor prescribed a diuretic and beta blocker. Since Leslie was 50 pounds overweight and had a constant craving for sugar, she was told to watch her caloric intake and try to eat a balanced diet. No one ever explained what a balanced diet was in terms of carbohydrates, fats, proteins, calories and essential fatty acids. She continued to gain weight and her blood pressure remained high. Her doctor increased her blood pressure medication. By this time the side effects of the medicine were making her uncomfortable. She began losing minerals because of the diuretic, and the beta blockers slowed her heart rate to the point where she was constantly tired. The mineral loss caused an imbalance in her electrolytes (sodium, potassium, magnesium and calcium) leading to a further rise in blood pressure.

Note: When blood pressure is artificially lowered by medication, the body tries to rebalance itself by two natural substances, renin and angiotensin. Both lessen the effect of the diuretic, and then the doctor raises the dosage.

Realizing that the medication was not helping her, she sought a more effective method and came to me for a consultation. I explained how blood pressure could be brought down to normal levels by losing weight and taking natural herbal diuretics and vitamins. She lost weight on a high protein, low carbohydrate diet. Herbal diuretics rid her body of excess fluid, and vitamins and minerals replaced nutrients lost from taking blood pressure medication. Leslie is now 30 pounds lighter, and her blood pressure is down to 128 over 76.

CANCER

A 47-year-old overweight woman, who led a stressful lifestyle and was a heavy smoker, discovered a lump in her left breast during a monthly self-examination. Her internist referred her to an oncologist who ordered a biopsy which showed a malignancy in a three centimeter size tumor. The doctors performed a lumpectomy, followed by radiation and chemotherapy.

She suffered hair loss, extreme nausea, vomiting, loss of appetite and extreme dryness in her mouth leading to painful sores. She lost so much weight that she became weakened. At this point she felt the side effects were so horrendous and painful that she opted to discontinue conventional therapy.

After reading an article in a health magazine which described options in cancer treatment, she made some inquiries and contacted me. The first thing I advised was a high complex carbohydrate diet and the elimination of all animal type foods except fish. Specific herbs were recommended to enhance her decreased appetite. Supplements to enhance liver function were incorporated.

A detoxification program was initiated to eliminate toxic materials from the cancer cells that had been destroyed by chemotherapy and radiation. Four glasses of carrot juice daily from organically grown carrots supplied digestive enzymes and high amounts of organic Beta carotene. Pancreatic enzymes were also employed to destroy cancer cells. Antioxidant nutrients used were high amounts of Vitamins A, C and E along with selenium, glutathione, N-Aceytl cysteine and methionine. Laetrile (Vitamin B17) was utilized in the further destruction of cancer cells. Daily imagery and meditation were incorporated into her lifestyle.

Tumor marker testing was performed periodically to check levels of existing cancer cells. The latest test showed the elimination of all cancer cells in her body. Further testing by AMAS (Anti Malignant Antibody in Serum) showed normal levels.

This program is effective only if patients realize their total day and even part of the night must be devoted to the treatment. Ongoing philosophical therapy is strengthening patient's character to enable her to cope with the everyday adversities of life.

A 54-year-old VDT operator developed a high fever, weight loss, nausea, diarrhea and extreme lethargy. She was diagnosed with terminal pancreatic cancer. Chemotherapy was prescribed for six months followed by heavy doses of radiation. She was informed that her chances of survival were very low and the best she could hope for was to live out the year. Note: Pancreatic cancer is the most dangerous of all cancers, with a five-year survival rate of only one percent.

The woman felt she had been given a death sentence and came to me in such a severe state of depression that I had to utilize all my former experience in counseling depressed people to assure her that with natural healing she could exorcise this dread disease from her body. Initial treatment was metabolic therapy, composed of pancreatic enzymes, coffee enemas, carrot juice, Laetrile, a supplements program and a special diet tailored to fit her specific autonomic nervous system type. She was of the sympathetic type (high energy and fast oxidizer). Her diet consisted of complex carbohydrates, with digestive enzymes added, in order not to overuse her own pancreatic enzymes.

The patient's appetite increased and she started to gain weight slowly. Previous symptoms gradually disappeared and, through daily meditation and imagery, she has a renewed desire to live and function in society.

Carpal Tunnel Syndrome

Mary L., a beautician, developed such severe pains in the first three fingers of her right hand that she could no longer perform her job. She had been utilizing the same hand movements during her 15-year career as a beautician. Constant repetition of the same hand and wrist movements in any occupation promotes overextension of muscles, ligaments, tendons and nerves in the area, causing inflammation and pain.

Her internist prescribed prednisone. After she took the medication for six months, the carpal tunnel syndrome pain diminished somewhat but was not completely eliminated. She developed back pain and X-rays showed compression fractures of two vertebrae. This is one of the main side effects of prednisone since it slows the absorption of protein and calcium needed for strong bone structure. In her case, as millions of others, the side effects of medical treatment for one condition had brought on a more severe problem.

Mary had consulted me previously for a weight problem and asked me what could be done to eliminate the pain in her back and hand. An investigation into her past history, along with a hair analysis, revealed her heavy metal levels. Aluminum, lead and copper were so high that the readings were off the charts. These high levels were caused by the chemicals in the materials she used in the beauty parlor. The shop was improperly ventilated, exacerbating the mixture of the chemicals with carbon dioxide exhaled by the customers and staff.

I began a detoxification program immediately, and I told her to discontinue working for at least five to six weeks to try to eliminate the heavy metals from her system. The detoxification program consisted of a liver flush, blood cleansing herbs and sulfur containing amino acids with silymarin (milk thistle) to strengthen the liver, which is the body's main detoxifying organ. Other supplements were also incorporated in order to rebuild her immune system. She decided to discontinue the prednisone and use Microcrystalline Hydroxyapatite Concentrate (Bone Builder) to rebuild her bone structure. Vitamins B2 and B6 helped reduce the accumulation of fluid and swelling in the carpal tunnel area of her fingers and wrist.

After six weeks, her back pain was totally gone and the carpal tunnel syndrome had lessened to such a degree that she was able to return to work. She now works in a shop with a better ventilation system to avoid having the condition return.

CATARACTS

At her annual eye examination, Flo B. was told the macular area of her eye was degenerating and that it was a normal part of the aging process. She was also told the lens in each eye was starting to degenerate and would eventually lead to cataracts. The degeneration had not affected her eyesight. There are two types of macular degeneration, wet (bleeding) and dry. Hers was the wet type which is more serious. To stop the bleeding, laser surgery was recommended. A side effect of this procedure is loss of macular cells which do not regenerate. She was also told she would require cataract surgery in the future.

Note: The lens protects the macula from solar rays which may destroy retinal cells. In cases of macular degeneration, it is better to retain one's natural lens as long as possible.

I instead recommended specific supplements to enhance the rebuilding of her existing macular cells. These included zinc, selenium, Vitamin E, calcium and glutathione which act as antioxidants in cleansing toxic debris from the eye. I also gave her the herbs eyebright and bilberry and Vitamin B2 (riboflavin) which also cleanse toxic debris from the eye by activating the liver to cleanse this toxic debris fom the blood which would eventually migrate to the eyes.

Most conditions of macular degeneration cannot be reversed, but through the natural healing process, they can be arrested. Her next examination with the ophthalmologist revealed the bleeding had stopped and the clouding of the lens of her eye had diminished. The doctor was astounded with the results and the patient is extremely happy.

Cholesterol

A male nurse, head of a surgical department, had a history of high cholesterol (262) and high triglycerides (255). Two years prior to seeing me, he suffered a coronary occlusion. Cholesterol lowering medication had been prescribed, but nothing had been given to lower his triglycerides. Although his cholesterol readings were brought down while on medication, the side effects (liver problems, depression, lowered libido and headaches) upset and frightened him so much that he decided to stop taking the medicine. His cholesterol returned to 262, and the triglycerides stayed the same.

A nutritional cholesterol and triglyceride lowering program was initiated. This included fish oil, high fiber intake, a high protein low carbohydrate diet, niacin, chromium picolinate and garlic. In a three week period his cholesterol dropped to 185 and triglycerides to 115. No side effects were encountered. His physician was overwhelmed that the levels were reduced so quickly without medication. He has remained on the program and, since then, his triglycerides and cholesterol have stabilized at normal levels.

CHRONIC FATIGUE SYNDROME

Nancy Pollack, M.S., Psychotherapist, Korean Martial Arts Black Belt, suffered from chronic fatigue syndrome and Candida albicans. Her energy level was extremely low and denied her the ability to fulfill her obligations at work. By noon she was completely exhausted and had to return home to rest.

The candida caused highly poisonous toxins to enter her bloodstream and evoke multiple infectious syndromes. This condition was so debilitating that she considered giving up her job and entering the hospital.

She was referred to me and immediately taken off all sugars, yeast, fermented foods, dairy products, mushrooms, grains and caffeine. High amounts of specific supplements were recommended to stimulate her immune system to rid her body of the candida and eliminate the chronic fatigue.

The debilitating effects of chronic fatigue syndrome and systemic candida can continue for years unless the cause is addressed. Most patients suffering from these ailments are deficient in the transfer of oxygen on a cellular level. Therefore oxygenating nutrients such as germanium, hydrogen peroxide 35 percent food grade, ozone therapy and DMG were utilized.

She was also instructed to drink distilled water and put on an exercise program. Daily meditation also added to her recovery. She is now fully recovered, back to work, and is leading a normal life.

CYSTITIS

Mollie R. had ongoing bouts of chronic cystitis that were not being helped by orthodox methods, and she sought alternative therapy. Her mother and older sister had the same problem. All received antibiotic therapy which relieved the problem temporarily, but caused side effects such as vaginal yeast infections.

The purpose of antibiotic therapy is to destroy the bacteria causing the initial problem, but they also destroy the remaining friendly bacteria necessary for proper balance. *The word "antibiotic" means against life, so it seems quite strange to use such a highly toxic and dangerous drug except for life-threatening conditions.*

When she first consulted me, she was unhappy, anxious and frustrated with her previous therapy. Cystitis is usually caused from an overalkaline environment of the bladder. In other words, urine should be in an acid state in order to destroy unfriendly bacteria in the area. Supplements recommended to acidify her urine were Vitamin C, cranberry juice and apple cider vinegar. Foods leading to an alkaline state in the body were removed from her diet temporarily. These included fruits, vegetables, millet, buckwheat, Brazil nuts and coconut. I also suggested she avoid highly spiced foods, such as mustard, ketchup and alcohol.

She had no symptoms as long as she kept her urine at the correct level by following the revised diet and taking the recommended supplements. On a two-week vacation, she went off the diet and neglected taking her supplements and the symptoms returned. This convinced her to adhere to the program. I stress to my patients that conviction is the byword to success and, without conviction, a human being will constantly repeat a deleterious lifestyle leading to failure.

Her mother and sister were appalled at first when she discontinued conventional therapy, but when they saw how well she was doing, both went on my program with excellent results.

DEPRESSION

Ruth P., a 58-year-old woman who suffered from constant depression, lethargy and digestive disturbances was referred to a psychiatrist by her family physician. He found that a chemical imbalance was turning her into a manic depressive. Diagnosis was made on the basis of visual and oral analysis, rather than by laboratory testing. She was given antidepressants to rebalance her brain chemistry. She took them for two months and returned to the psychiatrist for further evaluation. Her condition did not improve, and he increased her medication. Again no blood tests were ordered. The medication increased her feelings of lethargy and fatigue.

She was referred to me by a friend who had had a similar problem. In consultation I described the testing that would be necessary to determine the actual chemical imbalance. The primary test is a BEAM (Brain Electrical Activity Mapping) test. It is a stress type electroencephalogram. A blood test would also be necessary to evaluate the levels of neurotransmitters and amino acids which allow for the accurate transport of messages from brain neuron to brain neuron.

We incorporated a simple electrical stimulating system of the brain which energizes the areas not receiving their full complement of neurotransmitters. This was performed at the Brain Bio Center in Princeton, N.J. In addition, her amino acids levels were off to such a degree as to cause malfunctioning of key receptor sites in the brain, specifically levels of the neurotransmitters acetylcholine and dopamine.

I recommended supplementation which brought her amino acid levels up to normal, and also enhanced neurotransmitter activity. These allowed Ruth to regain her emotional stability. She is now able to cope with life in a contented manner and her digestive problems have disappeared.

DIABETES

A 64-year-old part-time secretary and amateur violinist gained 50 pounds over a 30-year period. She suffered from tingling and numbness in her toes which she disregarded until new symptoms arose. These were extreme thirst and hunger, sugar cravings and constant urination. Upon casual conversation with a diabetic co-worker, she realized she had a problem and made an appointment with an endocrinologist. The only tests performed were urinalysis and fasting blood sugar and the medical doctors discovered she had adult onset diabetes #2. This occurs in older people and is much different from juvenile diabetes where insulin is not produced at all.

Her physician did not suggest insulin testing so it was never determined how much insulin she produced. Without this knowledge, insulin shots were prescribed. Her blood sugar decreased and symptoms were relieved but she suffered side effects of thickening of the blood, accompanied by slight occluding of the arteries, increased sugar craving and more weight gain. Insulin testing was still not performed and her dosage was increased. The only dietary advice given was to eat a balanced diet.

In a national health magazine, she read an article dealing with adult onset diabetes. It mentioned the dangerous side effects of insulin and showed how adult onset diabetes can be treated through a process of a strict high protein, low carbohydrate diet, accompanied by the elimination of all sugars and processed foods and the addition of specific nutrients.

Soon after she saw me. She was delighted to learn that blood sugar could be lowered naturally and the insulin made more effective by natural methods. A high protein, low carbohydrate diet was immediately instituted, along with the aid of supplements. These were chromium picolinate, L-Alanine, zinc, magnesium, biotin, pyridoxol alphaketaglutarate.

Under my supervision, she lost a significant amount of weight. Insulin was no longer necessary. All original symptoms and side effects of therapy have disappeared and she is delighted that she no longer has to give herself insulin injections. Her co-worker was so impressed that she is now in a similar program.

Note: In certain cases of adult onset diabetes, blood sugar lowering medications are used. These medications increase your chance of a heart attack by two and a half times.

Miriam J., a lawyer, was diagnosed with adult onset diabetes at the age of 39. Her symptoms were loss of appetite, weight loss, craving for sugar, excessive thirst and frequency of urination. Blood tests performed by an endocrinologist revealed a blood sugar of 376. Medication recommended to lower blood sugar was not effective and insulin was recommended. Miriam was against taking insulin because of her sister's experience with its side effects which was atherosclerosis that had led to heart failure. She was never told to stop consuming fruit and fruit juices which exacerbated her condition because of the ineffectiveness of her insulin.

The first thing I suggested was that she stop eating most carbohydrates and raise the level of protein in her diet. I also recommended a strenuous exercise program which is one of the most effective ways to lower high blood sugar. Activating muscles utilizes high amounts of sugar, thereby lowering the amount in the bloodstream. A half mile walk following each meal was also incorporated for the sole purpose of lowering an increase in blood sugar following meals.

I emphasized the importance of the diet and exercise more so than supplements in her case, which was effective. She also lost weight which was necessary, and since most carbohydrates were eliminated, her need for insulin was reduced and her blood sugar eventually came down to normal levels.

DIGESTIVE DISTURBANCES

After years of flatulence, burping and heartburn, Norma G., a housewife, saw her family doctor to try to ascertain what the problem was. The doctor could not find anything wrong clinically and prescribed an over the counter antacid. This was totally ineffective and she returned to the doctor who then ordered an upper and lower GI, both of which were negative. He never investigated her diet, but recommended further testing including colonoscopy.

Her symptoms were worsening and she decided to investigate another way to handle the problem. She had heard of nutritionists but did not know exactly what they did. She picked up one of my cards in a health food store and made an appointment. I am always appalled when patients tell me their physicians have not addressed their diets because most digestive problems are easily eliminated by removing offending foods.

The chief cause of bowel disturbances in our society is that most people eat the same foods day after day. Individual metabolisms are developed toward specific foods that are compatible with a person's unique digestive process. They must ingest only the specific foods that can be broken down in the system to the tiniest molecules in order to prevent them from becoming an offending agent. If a person eats the same foods daily and is allergic to one or more of them, he or she will have an allergic reaction which will cause the digestive problem. Eating the same food daily does not give the digestive process time to recoup from the offending foods. However this is never pointed out to patients with digestive problems. Instead they are told to take medicine or have surgical procedures which do nothing for the initial cause of poor digestion.

Listening to Norma, I surmised that she was a fast oxidizer which means she metabolizes food at such a fast rate her stomach is empty most of the time. This allows an overactive acid state in the stomach because there is not enough food available to be digested. She had been following a high complex carbohydrate vegetarian-type diet, thinking it would lead to better health. She had learned about this type of diet from reading magazines and watching television and listening to talk shows on the radio. Although this is a healthy diet in some cases, it is very generalized and does not apply to all individuals, yet many individuals apply it to themselves. In her case, therefore, a higher fat and protein type diet would remain in her stomach longer, absorbing the digestive acids and also preventing her from being hungry as often. A protein, fat type diet would be more filling and would prevent her from consuming so many carbohydrates. In addition to the dietary changes, supplements were incorporated into her program, including acidophilus, chlorophyll and aloe vera gel.

She now follows a diet that is metabolically correct for her, has lost weight and her problems have disappeared. Although complex carbohydrate diets are very much in vogue presently, they are not right for everybody. All diets should be metabolically tailored for each individual's unique digestive system.

Dry Eyes

A 68-year-old man constantly complained of dryness in both eyes. His internist suggested he purchase over-the-counter artificial tears. These gave temporary relief, but the problem persisted. The internist then believed the condition was due to an autoimmune disorder and prescribed prednisone. When this did not work, he was referred to an ophthalmologist who recommended sealing the lacrimal ducts so that that the small amounts of tears produced would not be wasted.

The patient became upset with the prognosis and was referred to me. I explained that his insufficient tears were caused by his body's inability to produce a specific prostaglandin which was needed to eliminate the inflammatory process in that area. Sufficient amounts of essential fatty acids are necessary for that prostaglandin to work efficiently. In his case, the essential fatty acids were depleted.

Essential fatty acids are derived from oils such as GLA from flax-seed oil, borage oil or fish oils. We used these oils, along with other supplements, to eliminate inflammatory problems. After two months on the regime, his dry eye problem was totally eliminated and his tear ducts and tear glands worked efficiently.

FIBROIDS

A 33-year-old computer operator that I was treating for M.S. casually mentioned to me that her periods were heavy and lasted seven days, with severe cramping. Bleeding was so heavy that she became anemic and was prescribed B12 and Iron. I referred her to a gynecologist who discovered a large fibroid in her uterus. He recommended antihormonal medication for a trial period of three months. After that time she was re-examined. The fibroid had not significantly changed and her symptoms remained active.

He recommended a hysterectomy because she was losing so much blood that her life could be in danger. Since she was knowledgeable about health alternatives, she asked what I would recommend. I explained that 50 percent of women have fibroids, and they usually disappear at menopause. However, she was several years away from menopause.

Proper diet and supplements to deactivate estrogen can shrink fibroid tumors. I recommended that she eliminate foods that stimulate estrogen production—along with sugars and fats which cause production of adipose (fat) tissue which stores estrogen. I gave her supplements to strengthen the effectiveness of her liver to neutralize the active form of estrogen.

Within three periods, most of her symptoms had disappeared. She returned to the gynecologist who was amazed how much the fibroids had shrunk.

GALLSTONES

Four hours after ingesting a heavy meal at Thanksgiving, a 42-year-old mother of two young children experienced vomiting, fever and severe upper abdominal pain radiating to her upper right shoulder. She was in such severe distress that she was rushed to the hospital where diagnostic tests revealed a gallbladder containing many medium size gallstones. Backup of bile exerts extreme pressure on the gallbladder and liver. A cholecystectomy (removal of the gallbladder) was recommended by the doctors as the only possible treatment. She fled the hospital when her doctor said, "Cut her open."

The patient chose to consult a natural healing practitioner instead. When I saw her, I immediately began a gallbladder flush (olive oil and lemon juice). The next morning she observed several gallstones in her stool, and pain and other symptoms had disappeared. She was instructed to follow a low fat, low sugar diet to prevent the problem from recurring.

Gallstones are a metabolic problem with the liver. Removing the gallbladder does not correct the basic problem which will eventually damage the liver and destroy the body. The patient adhered to the diet and a nutritional regimen for strengthening the liver with specific herbs. The problem has not recurred.

HEADACHES

Susan L., a 44-year-old woman, had suffered from chronic headaches since adolescence. A series of lengthy, costly diagnostic procedures including CAT scans and an MRI were performed to rule out malignancies. Prescription painkillers were recommended and temporarily relieved the headaches. However they returned with a vengeance and increased doses of the medication became less and less effective. She changed doctors and different painkillers were prescribed which were even less effective than those taken previously. None of the doctors she consulted investigated the possibility of food allergies or nutrient imbalances.

Susan finally decided upon a new course of action which was to consult a nutritionally-oriented doctor. A series of food allergy tests and special blood tests performed on the white cells showed her system was severely deficient in protein. Her diet had consisted mainly of complex carbohydrates. In addition, certain foods caused an allergic reaction which lead directly to her headaches.

The foods causing the allergic reaction were eliminated from her diet, and higher amounts of protein were recommended. Nutritional supplements included niacin (vasodilator), feverfew (herb), anti-inflammatory prostaglandin, magnesium (muscle relaxant) and B complex.

The headaches disappeared in 24 hours. They do not return unless she becomes lax about her diet or neglects to take maintenance doses of her supplements.

Heart Disease

A 55-year-old male chef noticed shortness of breath upon exertion, plus slight pain in his upper chest and lower jaw, accompanied with numbness and slight pain radiating down his left arm. His family practitioner examined him and performed an electrocardiogram and referred him to a cardiologist. Cardiac catheterization revealed a 95 percent blockage in the main coronary artery. A bypass procedure was recommended. In fact, he was told that the doctor would not be responsible for his life unless this was done within two weeks.

Although he was terrified by this pronouncement, he had previous positive experiences with alternative healing and decided to follow that route. Chelation therapy was recommended. Through a series of intravenous solutions the arteries are cleansed of all plaque and debris. The solution consists of amino acid chelators with added vitamins and minerals to replace those lost during the chelation process.

Lifestyle changes included cessation of smoking and drinking alcoholic beverages and the elimination of fatty and sugary type foods. After ten chelation treatments, he had no more symptoms. Twenty further treatments were necessary to fulfil the requirements of chelation standards. Maintenance chelation was utilized yearly to insure arterial health.

A nutritional program of vitamins, minerals and amino acids was incorporated to keep the arteries clear and his blood at the proper viscosity. Digestive imbalances were addressed.

It has now been three years since his initial chelation therapy and the patient has remained stable. Further catheterizaton tests were not employed because of dangerous side effects which, in certain cases, can lead to death. Instead, thallium stress testing was utilized. Not only has he lost weight and stopped smoking and drinking, but in three years he has not had a recurrence of the original problem.

An 80-year-old female was told to have a quadruple bypass and replacement of the aortic valve. Even though her physician said she would die if the procedures were not done immediately, she decided against the surgery. On a person of this age, these surgical procedures could have a failure rate of 98 percent, but this was not explained to her.

Due to a strong belief in natural healing methods, she opted to follow my program. Initially, a weight loss program was instituted to reduce pressure on her arteries and heart. Symptoms of fatigue, breathlessness and swelling of lower extremities began to dissipate.

I gave her supplements to lessen the effects of her blocked arteries and her weakened heart muscle and to strengthen her aortic valve. When surgery replaces the aortic valve by a synthetic valve, the patient must stay on blood thinners for life, and they may worsen the original condition.

She was also given nutrients that not only eliminate symptoms but also rebuild degenerated tissue: CoEnzyme Q10, hawthorne (herb), Vitamin C, magnesium oritate, L-Carnitine, germanium, bromelain and garlic.

Symptoms of fatigue, breathlessness and swelling of her lower extremities gradually faded. Nine months later she celebrated her 81st birthday. All symptoms have now dissipated, and she is leading an active life.

A bus driver, George W., had recurrent chest pains radiating down his left arm and to his chin. His physician said it was indigestion and would eventually disappear. When the symptoms worsened, he returned to his doctor, who then ordered an angiogram to test for heart function. This test, cardiac catheterization, is a 100 percent invasive procedure with the dangerous side effect of possible death. The test revealed blockage in two arteries, 95 percent in one and 90 percent in the other.

George was told that he should have a balloon angioplasty immediately in order to survive. Since he was frightened and concerned about his life, he agreed. During this procedure, a catheter with a balloon attached is threaded to the blocked part of the artery and the balloon is inflated to compress the blockage onto the sides of the artery, hopefully enlarging the blocked area to renewed blood flow. He was not informed that 35 percent of patients undergoing this procedure have a recurrence in six months.

When his symptoms returned, he would not undergo the same procedure again. After reading an article in a health magazine and learning that such blockages of coronary arteries can be reversed through natural methods, he came to see me.

I explained that by simply changing his diet, the condition could be reversed. Changes included elimination of all animal foods and foods containing processed sugar. This is the type diet proved successful by the late Nathan Pritikin. Specific supplements were included, including Vitamin C, niacin, bromelain, fish oils, pantothene, CoEnzyme Q10 and L-Carnitine.

This proved effective, and his symptoms subsided in two weeks. After a year of following the program conscientiously, George feels better than ever and told me his wife was complaining that he was too active.

Hemorrhoids

A 39-year-old police officer assigned to traffic direction at a major intersection, noticed bright red blood in the toilet bowl following a bowel movement. He also had a protrusion in his anal area. He was terrified and made an appointment with a proctologist who found hemorrhoids and recommended surgery, which is extremely painful. It also takes two to three weeks following the surgery for the patient to have a bowel movement without pain. In fact, the initial bowel movements after the surgery are so painful that many patients live in great fear of them and try to avoid eliminating, causing a backup of toxins into the system.

Hoping to avoid surgery, he contacted me. I explained that hemorrhoids are nothing more than weakened veins in the anal area. If the walls of these veins can be strengthened, they can return to their normal size, allowing bowel movements that would not place undue stress on the weakened veins. These protrusions, external hemorrhoids, can usually be gently pushed back into the anal area, and the problem of bleeding disappears. But this can be effective only if the cause of the problem, which is constipation or diarrhea, is first treated.

I investigated the officer's diet and made suggestions for immediate changes. His diet lacked sufficient amounts of fiber to add bulk to the feces. This caused frequent small bowel movements which overstressed the anal area. I also recommended that he apply a mixture of milk of magnesia and witch hazel in equal parts to the anal area after every bowel movement and before retiring. Supplements included rutin (bioflavanoid) to strengthen the venous area, pantothene and bromelain as anti-inflammatories for inflammation and pain.

After the hemorrhoids receded, the milk of magnesia and witch hazel applications were replaced with Vitamin E oil following bowel movements and before retiring.

Note: Since the officer's job entails standing on concrete eight hours a day, gravity tends to proliferate hemorrhoids. This applies to all occupations where people stand constantly. I recommended he resole his work shoes with crepe soles to lessen the impact of standing on concrete. The patient adhered to the program 100 percent and has fully recovered.

IMPOTENCE

A 27-year-old stockbroker—married two years—was anxious to become a father, but started to suffer from loss of libido and an inability to sustain an erection while making love to his wife. The situation was extremely frustrating, especially since they wanted a child. A urologist examined him and tested his sperm count and penile blood pressure. All tests proved negative and the urologist could find no physiological reasons for his impotence. He was referred to a psychiatrist for antidepressant medication and psychotherapy. Six months later there was no improvement. He and his wife were upset and frustrated with the lack of success and the time and money invested.

They had been conditioned to believe in orthodox medicine and did not seek alternative methods until a friend confided that I had treated him for a similar problem. An investigation of his nutritional status and health habits revealed he was smoking, drinking alcohol and coffee and that his diet consisted mainly of fast food products and processed sugar. He was not exercising because he claimed he didn't have the time and was 35 pounds overweight. None of the three physicians he had consulted ever investigated his diet or lifestyle.

The program I designed for him consisted of reversing the negative aspects of his lifestyle. Happy hour was replaced with a visit to a gym. He stopped smoking and reduced caffeine consumption. I gave him specific herbs and vitamins to regenerate his circulation and his libido. These included yohimbe, ginseng, Saw palmetto berries, damiana, a one-a-day vitamin/mineral combination, Vitamin E and zinc.

The program was extremely effective and proved that his original problem was not psychological or neurological, but simply a deficiency and imbalance in nutrients. At my last contact with him, he happily told me his wife had given birth to twins.

INSOMNIA

An air traffic controller on shift work experienced difficulty falling and remaining asleep. His primary physician examined him and could not find a physical reason for his problem. Blood tests, electrocardiogram, chest X-ray and blood pressure were within normal limits. The doctor sent him to a sleep disorder clinic where he stayed overnight for further testing. They found some discrepancies in his REM sleep and beta waves and recommended medication to help him sleep. The medication was not particularly effective and he noticed some effect on his concentration and mental acuity, so necessary for his responsible job.

A change in his medication was suggested, but he decided to explore a different method of treatment and consulted me. An investigation of his lifestyle, diet and symptoms led me to believe his body was in an acid state. Sleeping is predicated on the body being in an alkaline (anabolic) condition. This allows the body cells to rebuild. When the body is in an acid (catabolic) state, alpha waves are disturbed, promoting wakefulness.

Note: The body's acid/alkaline states change during the course of the day. The body works on two 12 hour phases. During the catabolic phase, the cells break down to produce energy, and the body is in an acid state. During the anabolic state, the body repairs itself. This occurs while sleeping, and if the body is too acid at that time, sleep patterns will be disturbed.

In order to alkalinize his body, we changed his diet to alkaline-producing foods and supplements including green magma (powdered greens), Vitamin E, zinc, iron, chromium and molybdenum. This regime is usually foolproof unless physiological or psychological reasons are present.

Since this person was on shift work, his circadian rhythms also had to be considered. These rhythms prevent the body from entering an alkaline state during daylight hours. Since at times he had to sleep during the day, I recommended melatonin which is needed for relaxing and has no effect on concentration. Melatonin, a precursor to seratonin, the body's natural tranquilizer, is produced during daylight, and he was not producing his own when he worked nights.

His sleep patterns have improved and he feels more confident about the responsibilities of his job.

KIDNEY STONES

Jeffrey B., an electrical construction worker, awakened during the night with severe lower back pain. He was in such agony that he called emergency medical services who took him to the hospital where he was admitted and given painkillers. Following a urologic consultation and X-rays, a small stone blocking the left ureter was discovered. This caused urine to back up into the kidney, leading to severe pressure and pain.

The urologist recommended he drink large amounts of fluid to increase urinary output and hopefully flush the stone through the urinary tract. This was effective and the stone was eliminated, but nothing was suggested as to the cause of the problem or what could be done to prevent a future recurrence. Analysis of the stone showed it was the product of an overabundance of calcium.

He was interested in learning how to avoid forming more stones and came for a consultation. I explained how excess calcium in the bloodstream has to be broken into a soluble form to avoid collecting in the tubules of the kidneys where it undergoes a process of accumulation, forming a stone. The stone either blocks the kidney at that point or is released through the ureter where it can become stuck, causing extreme pressure and pain.

Further investigation determined that his system was too alkaline, which led to the insolubility of his calcium. I changed his diet incorporating higher acid-forming foods and supplementation with apple cider vinegar, betaine hydrochloric acid and glutamic acid to aid in the breakdown of calcium to a soluble form. In a follow-up visit, he mentioned that the pain in his arthritic knee had disappeared, along with muscle cramps in his lower legs that often disturbed his sleep. The reason for these positive side effects is that calcium was able to be transported to areas where it is effective rather than being stored as calcium deposits.

LEG CRAMPS

Genevieve R., a housewife, complained of cramping in the muscles of both legs when she attempted to get out of bed in the morning. Her husband had to massage them vigorously and help her walk for at least ten minutes to regain some circulation to alleviate the pain.

For the past several years, Genevieve had given up orthodox therapy for her ailments because of the side effects of medicine and treatments which usually exacerbated her problems. When she consulted me, I explained that leg cramps (intermittent claudication) was basically a problem of improper balance between contraction and expansion of the muscles. Usually this is due to an imbalance of electrolytes (potassium, magnesium, calcium and sodium).

I recommended a hair analysis to check mineral imbalances and ratios in her body. The results showed she was extremely low in calcium and potassium which imbalanced magnesium and sodium ratios. It took several weeks to adjust the ratios since each person's system is different and it takes an expert to tailor the proper mineral replacement amounts. When balance was effected, her pain was relieved. She has followed the program conscientiously, and the leg cramps have not returned.

MENOPAUSE

A 53-year-old housewife suffered from hot flashes that disrupted her sleep. After falling and injuring her back, X-rays taken were negative for fractures, but did show slight bone loss in the long bones, the beginning of osteoporosis. Periodic heart palpitations frightened and disturbed her. After visiting her primary physician on her H.M.O. plan, she was referred to a gynecologist who recommended estrogen replacement therapy. The physician said the benefits (relief of hot flashes, vaginal dryness and arrested bone loss) would outweigh the risks of breast lumps, blood clots, weight gain and the possibility of uterine cancer.

She was not the type of person who believed in taking medication unless she was seriously ill. After weighing the benefits against the risks, she sought alternative therapy. There she learned that, by adding specific foods and nutrients, estrogen could be supplied to her body in a safe manner. Existing small amounts of estrogen residing in her adrenal glands and fat tissue were used to replace the estrogen that was no longer supplied by her ovaries.

Her program consisted of a diet of high estrogen-type foods, brewers yeast, sunflower seeds, alfalfa, wheat germ and estrogen-producing nutrients, including high amounts of folic acid, PABA, boron and the herbal combination Change of Life.

Her hot flashes diminished, her heart palpitations ceased and X-rays showed that her loss of bone had been arrested.

MULTIPLE SCLEROSIS

A 49-year-old former model living in New York City suffered from periodic bouts of multiple sclerosis. She had been treated with Prednisone, the orthodoxy's only available therapy for MS. This treatment did nothing for her condition, but had serious side effects, including swelling of her arms and legs, problems with the retina of her eyes and adrenal dysfunction. After the patient went for a second opinion and the same procedure was recommended, she opted for natural healing methods and contacted me in April of 1990.

I questioned her about her symptoms and lifestyle and determined that immediate changes were necessary. I instructed her to stop smoking and give up caffeinated beverages, specifically coffee and cola drinks. Through the process of a rotation diet, I was able to determine what foods she was allergic to and should stop eating. Additional dietary changes such as elimination of sugars, animal fats and dairy products proved to be successful.

I recommended these nutrients: Calcium EAP, essential fatty acids, Evening primrose oil (GLA), Vitamin B12 (for improved nerve function), octocosonal (for muscle control) and Vitamin E, along with monounsaturated vegetable oils for repair of her nerve sheath. High amounts of antioxidants were used to stimulate her immune system to such a degree as to discourage another outbreak of the disease. Light exercise and sunning were also incorporated into the program.

In a month and a half, the patient contacted me to report that she was able to walk in high heels without pain. She has now fully resumed a normal life without the constant worry, pain and stress which is associated with the disease. She calls me periodically to thank me for her renewed health and continues to progress to the degree where it is difficult for her to remember her disability.

OBESITY

Steven G., a 35-year-old systems engineer with continuous weight problems since adolescence constantly tried various weight loss programs. He always regained what he lost, and more, due to losing lean body muscle mass caused by high carbohydrate, low protein diets.

He was put on a high protein, low carbohydrate diet and exercise program and immediately started to lose weight. After a two month period, he lost 20 pounds which brought him down to a healthy weight for his height and age. He had no problems with the diet, felt fully satiated at meals and did not feel hungry between meals.

Complex carbohydrates were reintroduced into the diet on a staggered schedule. He has remained at his desired weight, has more energy and has regained lean body muscle mass.

Note: In some cases, nutritional supplements are recommended to raise the metabolic level in order to enhance the burning of fat.

PROSTATE ENLARGEMENT

A 62-year-old stage actor awakened several times a night to urinate. Lack of sleep caused his health to deteriorate and the pressure on his bladder while acting interfered with his career. He did not realize what the problem was until he tried to relieve himself at night and he could not release any urine at all. He immediately consulted a urologist, who performed a digital examination and discovered that his prostate had enlarged so much it completely blocked the flow of urine from his bladder. Catheterization was needed to relieve the pressure. The urologist then recommended a prostate operation, a T.U.R.P. procedure (trans urethral resection of the prostate).

When the patient learned about the side effects of the operation, he consulted me for a second opinion. Natural healing methods consisted of supplements C, zinc, Saw palmetto (herb), manganese, Vitamin E and three amino acids, L-Glycine, L-Glutamine and L-Alanine.

After following the program for two months, the prostate shrank to almost normal size. Arising at night decreased from five times to once and he was able to act without distress.

A 64-year old retired police officer was informed by his physician at a yearly checkup that his prostate was overly enlarged. He had no symptoms, but was told to have the prostate removed due to the possibility of a future malignancy. The patient did not understand why such a grave operation should be done when he felt good and did not wake up at night to urinate.

When the patient contacted me, he was in an overly active, anxious state. He brought copies of all tests and procedures that had been performed. After analyzing the information, I explained the latest holistic method used to shrink this type of prostate enlargement, which is localized hyperthermia, a non-surgical procedure that is 90 percent effective. In addition specific nutrients are also recommended.

Hyperthermia is a system of electrically stimulating the prostate. Nodes are placed on the prostate, either through the rectum or through a catheter inserted in the penis. Electrical stimulation in the correct frequency produces low heat which shrinks the cells of the prostate. The procedure was effective and the patient was delighted that he did not have to endure the anxiety and trauma of surgery.

TINNITUS

Alfred J., a guitarist in a rock band, complained of ringing in his ears that was so annoying he was unable to sleep. He also noticed that his hearing had become impaired. Examination by an ear, nose and throat specialist and an audiologist revealed damage to the inner ear and small punctures of the ear drums. The only available treatment was delicate surgery with a low rate of success. After considering the pros and cons of the surgery he inquired about other treatment methods.

Due to lack of circulation in the inner ear, the area was deficient in energy and oxygen that should have been derived from his bloodstream. The most common reason for this is hypoglycemia (low blood sugar), which causes glucose levels to be so low that they can't energize all areas of the body. In order to compensate for this, circulation in certain areas, often the inner ear, is diminished, accompanied by nerve and tissue damage.

In order to regenerate the damaged tissue, it is important to address the low blood sugar problem and supply extra oxygen to the dysfunctional area. I changed his diet and incorporated the use of supplements, hydrogen peroxide, germanium and dimethyl glycine. The condition improved, but I explained that the loud music which caused the problem initially would probably lead to a recurrence. He is considering leaving the rock band and teaching and writing music.

These case histories are of serious and debilitating diseases that in most cases are not treated effectively by standard methods. The patients are determined to regain their health by actively participating in the program and taking responsibility for its outcome instead of relying on someone else.

Other patients with the same diseases and natural treatments do not always have similar success rates due to either the lack of experience of the therapist, not conscientiously abiding by the program or losing faith within themselves.

Patients and their families are appalled that the orthodoxy does not utilize a system of non-toxic therapy with no side effects. Fortunately the public is becoming enlightened about alternative methods and demanding more information.

A system that has to use medications with such toxic side effects to cure a disease seems to me to be highly antiquated in this age of high technology. It is anticipated that this method will eventually be replaced with a more intelligent form of therapy, one in which the patient will have more trust.

This book is not designed to denigrate the orthodox medical establishment. It is still definitely needed, especially in emergency situations and in areas of scientific investigation.

My purpose is to draw attention to the fact that alternative healing therapies and orthodox medicine can work together to ease pain and suffering.

ABOUT THE AUTHORS

Dr. Wagner has been a practicing nutritional medical counselor in the Philadelphia area for the past ten years. Patients seek his advice pertaining to various conditions and disabling diseases.

He is an excellent speaker and has been on the lecture circuit for several years.

Dr. Wagner is the former Assistant Director of the Pennsylvania branch of the American Nutritional Medical Association.

He has a Diploma in Nutrition from the Nutritionist's Institute of America, a Certificate from Dr. Jenk's School of Herbalism and Iridology, a Certificate from Wild Rose College of Natural Healing (Vitamins and Minerals).

Sylvia Goldfarb is a freelance writer, specializing in medical topics for newspapers, magazines and in-house publications. Some of the magazines her articles have appeared in include: *Today's O R Nurse, Natural Body And Fitness, Delaware Valley Magazine, Focus, Fodor's Guidebooks* and *Today's Secretary.*

She serves as a faculty member of the Philadelphia Writer's Conference, and teaches health care and lifestyle writing.

She is a graduate of Skidmore College and a member of the Author's Guild.